The Ichthyoses

The Ichthyoses

*Proceedings of the 2nd Annual Clinically Orientated Symposium of
The European Society for Dermatological Research*

EDITED BY

R. Marks and P. J. Dykes,
*Department of Medicine,
Welsh National School of Medicine,
Cardiff*

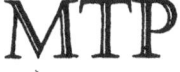

Published by
MTP Press Limited
St Leonard's House
St Leonardgate
Lancaster, England

ISBN 978-94-010-9853-3   ISBN 978-94-010-9851-9 (eBook)
DOI 10.1007/978-94-010-9851-9

Contents

CONTENTS

List of Contributors

Professor I. Anton-Lamprecht
University—Hautklinik
Heidelberg
West Germany

Dr. P. J. W. Ayres
S.R.P. Bioceutics
Walmer
Kent
England

Professor CL. Blanchet-Bardon
L'Hôpital St Louis
Paris
France

Professor R. Caputo
Universita di Milano
Italy

Dr. M. F. Cooper
University of Newcastle upon Tyne
England

Dr. M. G. Davies
Welsh National School of Medicine
Wales

Dr. P. J. Dykes
Welsh National School of Medicine
Wales

Dr. P. Fabbri
University of Florence
Italy

Dr. P. Frost
Mount Sinai Medical Center
Miami
USA

Dr. G. Gasparini
Universita di Milano
Italy

Professor F. Gianotti
Universita di Milano
Italy

Professor M. Greaves
Institute of Dermatology
London
England

Dr. P. S. Harper
Welsh National School of Medicine
Wales

Dr. R. Howell
Singleton Hospital
Swansea
Wales

Dr. M. Innocenti
Universita di Milano
Italy

Professor E. G. Jung
Hautklinik Stadt. Krankenanstalten
Heidelberg
West Germany

Miss C. S. King
Welsh National School of Medicine
Wales

Dr. R. Marks
Welsh National School of Medicine
Wales

Dr. D. McGibbon
University of Newcastle upon Tyne
England

Dr. J. D. Middleton
Inveresk Research International
Edinburgh
Scotland

LIST OF CONTRIBUTORS

Professor J. A. Milne
University of Glasgow
Scotland

Mr. S. Nicholls
Welsh National School of Medicine
Wales

Professor E. Panconesi
University of Florence
Italy

Dr. G. L. Peck
National Institutes of Health
Bethesda
USA

Dr. D. Peluchetti
Universita di Milano
Italy

Dr. C. Prottey
Unilever Research
Port Sunlight
England

Professor A. Puissant
L'Hôpital St. Louis
Paris
France

Dr. D. J. Reynolds
Welsh National School of Medicine
Wales

Mrs. M. E. Roberts
Inveresk Research International
Edinburgh
Scotland

Dr. W. Schalla
Freie Universität
Berlin
West Germany

Professor U. W. Schnyder
Univ. Hautklinik
Heidelberg
West Germany

Professor S. Shuster
University of Newcastle upon Tyne
England

Dr. D. Skerrow
University of Glasgow
Scotland

Professor G. Stuttgen
Freie Universität
Berlin
West Germany

Professor G. Swanbeck
Karolinska Institutet
Stockholm
Sweden

Dr. E. Waddington
University Hospital of Wales
Wales

Dr. E. J. Van Scott
Temple University
Philadelphia
USA

Dr. F. W. Yoder
National Institutes of Health
Bethesda
USA

Dr. R. J. Yu
Temple University
Philadelphia
USA

Foreword and Acknowledgements

The ichthyoses do not seem to have generated as much 'heat' in terms of dermatological research interest as have other common dermatoses such as psoriasis and allergic contact dermatitis. This is strange because insight into the tissue abnormalities in these disorders might not only benefit a large number of discomforted folk, but give important information concerning keratinization in general.

In recent years several groups have become aware of this problem and interesting work in this field is beginning to appear in the journals. The European Society for Dermatological Research felt that the ichthyoses would make a good topic for their second symposium and we considered ourselves lucky that it was agreed that this should be held in Cardiff. We hope that the meeting served to stimulate interest in the ichthyotic disorders and we trust that these proceedings will serve as a useful record of this event. We are extremely grateful to the enormous number of institutions, companies and individuals who helped make the meeting possible, and would like to record our sincere thanks to Eaton Laboratories in particular who made this publication possible. We are also grateful to:

Beecham Products Ltd.
Gist-Brocades nv.
Glaxo research Ltd.
Imperial Chemical Industries Ltd.
Knox Laboratories Ltd
E. Merck Ltd
Ortho Pharmaceutical Ltd.
Pharmacia (Great Britain) Ltd.
Schering Chemicals Ltd.
Stafford-Miller Ltd.

Stiefel Laboratories (U.K.) Ltd.
Tenovus
The Wellcome Trust
Guides Wales
Mid-Glamorgan Health Authority
South Glamorgan Health Authority
University Hospital of Wales
Wales Tourist Board
Welsh National School of Medicine

Introduction

On the way from a 'fish to philosopher' the evolution of the vertebrates had to solve the main problems of osmosis and respiration and in particular develop a protective outer surface for the individual organism — the SKIN!

The study of human EMBRYOLOGY does not give us insight into the evolutionary attempts resulting finally in the fascinating complex that constitutes human skin. The epidermis produces a horny envelope and this product of epidermal differentiation represents an almost ideal solution to the diverse problems faced by a surface structure. Flexibility, plasticity, sensitivity, provision of an osmotic barrier, protection against mechanical, chemical and microbial attack are some of its attributes.

However, PHYLOGENETIC studies provide examples showing overspecialization has drawbacks. The formation of scales, shells and carapaces in fishes, amphibia, reptiles and lower mammals are the best known 'cul-de-sacs' of evolution in keratinization.

The HORNY LAYER is the product of epidermal differentiation. A series of gene-controlled structural proteins and enzymes have to interact in a well-defined sequence. Keratinization will be impaired and the end product imbalanced if one or another of the gene products or the regulation of the stepwise process is lacking or faulty.

A series of such genetic defects of keratinization lead to a diffuse thickening and scaling of the horny layer, called the ICHTHYOSES. This is a heterogeneous group of diseases. The question arises as to whether one or another type of ichthyosis can be understood as a kind of atavism in which there is a regressive mutation simulating older phylogenetic attempts. Differentiation of the various clinical types of ichthyosis and ichthyosiform diseases; their treatment and genetic analysis, the pathological basis and biochemical characteristics, the functional alterations found and their possible implications; these are the topics of this symposium.

ERNEST G. JUNG
Mannheim, Germany
President, ESDR

Section 1
Pathogenetic Aspects

1

Metabolic Basis for Disturbed Keratinization in Ichthyosis and Other Diseases

E. J. VAN SCOTT and R. J. YU

Molecular structures of therapeutic agents now known to normalize disturbed keratinization in ichthyosis and other disorders of keratinization suggest that keratinization is normally modulated by certain α-hydroxy or α-keto acids. Evidence for this includes the demonstrated efficacy of topically applied α-hydroxy and α-keto acids in ichthyosis; the presence of ichthyotic skin in Refsum's disease, a disorder associated with failure of an α-hydroxylase; and preliminary findings that active forms of vitamin A acid may be hydroxylated derivatives.

IDENTITY OF KERATINIZATION ABNORMALITIES

The structural and functional properties of the cutaneous surface almost entirely are those of the stratum corneum, modified only slightly by influences of hair, sweat glands and sebaceous glands. The process of keratinization, consisting of the aggregate events by which the epidermis forms the stratum corneum, must be reviewed not only in context with epidermal syntheses of fibrous proteins, mucopolysaccharides and special compounds that modify the texture of the stratum corneum but with other epidermal attributes such as rates of stratum corneum production, and cohesiveness of stratum corneum cells, their hydrophilic and water-binding properties, their elasticity and pliability.

Many skin diseases secondarily affect the epidermis and thence the stratum corneum — events generally sequential to dermal inflammation. Such sequelae, however, should not be construed as representing diseases of keratinization even though keratinization is disturbed. Unfortunately, until the process of keratinization in its entirety is better understood, precise delineation of whether a cutaneous disease is or is not due to a primary defect in keratinization is not possible. But because of the desirability to establish and test hypotheses, it seems reasonable at this time to exclude as diseases of keratinization those disorders wherein disturbances in stratum corneum formation or shedding are consequent to other separably distinct pathologic events, whether epidermal, e.g. contact allergic dermatitis, or dermal, e.g. infectious exanthems. Few cutaneous afflictions therefore may be disorders primarily of keratinization. The following perhaps should be included as such:

Ordinary dry skin

Usually associated with advancing years, the condition is a frequent impairment of aging, although it may occur in younger years. Because it is worsened by excessive skin cleansing practices and by atmospheric low humidities, and because improvements are achieved by topical applications of preparations containing water or compounds that bind water, the cause of ordinary dry skin is thought to be due to deficient epidermal synthesis and retention of physiologic humectants. While this seems reasonable enough, it is probably too simplistic for a multiplicity of structural and functional attributes may be cited or conceptualized as distinguishing the skin surface of the younger from that of the older. Ordinary dry skin, however, does appear to be due to relative incompetence of some aspects of the process of keratinization.

Heritable ichthyoses

Comprised of several genetically transmitted diseases, these disorders appear to be valid disorders of keratinization. Although categorized into several types according to genetic patterns, clinical presentation and histological features, the ichthyoses are all related by the common denominator of defective cutaneous keratinization, which appears to be an isolated epidermal phenomenon insofar as hyperkeratinization of other epithelia does not occur.

Keratinization abnormalities caused by certain metabolic defects

While varying degrees of disturbed keratinization can occur with some diseases e.g. lymphomas, or with intake of certain drugs, e.g. triparanol, the relationship is variable and inconsistent. In two metabolic abnormalities, however, defective keratinization occurs quite consistently. The specificity of this association would seem to provide important clues regarding what the normal controls of keratinization might be. One metabolic abnormality is that of dietary vitamin

A deficiency wherein hyperkeratinization of epidermis and other epithelia occurs. The other metabolic defect is that encountered in Refsum's disease, an inherited neurological disorder biochemically characterized by accumulation of phytanic acid due to failure of tissue hydroxylases to initiate its degradation by α-hydroxylation. In this disease dry hyperkeratotic scaliness of the skin appears in variable degrees, reported to be at times sufficiently extreme to mimic ichthyosis. As in the ichthyoses, hyperkeratinization of other epithelia does not occur.

The paramount metabolic features that appear relevant to the entire foregoing group, and which may be applicable to normal physiological controls of keratinization, involves α- and perhaps β-hydroxy acids, the functionability of tissue hydroxylases, and possibly the interconvertibility of hydroxy and keto groups. These will be discussed further subsequently.

APPROACHES TO THERAPY OF DISORDERS IN KERATINIZATION

Two routes may be followed, either singly or simultaneously, for improving impaired physical properties and performance of the stratum corneum. One is by means that modify the stratum corneum after its formation by the epidermis, i.e. product alteration. The other is by means that modify the formation of stratum corneum, i.e. process alteration. Agents known today that can mediate these alterations are listed in Table 1.1.

Table 1.1 Pharmacologic agents that alter the stratum corneum or its formation

Product alteration	Process alteration
Hydrating agents	α-hydroxy acids
Water	α-keto acids
Glycerin	vitamin A metabolites
Propylene glycol	
Urea	
Pyroglutamic acid	
Sorbitol	
Keratolytics	
Alkalis	
Lithium salts	
Urea (>3M)	
Thiol compounds	

Hydration

The most commonly used means to modify the impaired stratum corneum have been those which enhance its hydration. Hydration is achieved by application of water *per se*, by application of chemical substances that attract or bind water, and/or by application of substances that retard evaporative water loss from the skin surface. The importance of water for maintenance of stratum corneum softness was formally demonstrated by the work of Blank a quarter century ago[1,2], although the principle seems to have been commercially appreciated years earlier in forms of water-containing lotions and cold creams that enjoyed rapid popularity.

The way in which water softens the stratum corneum appears to be performed at a rather macroscopic level, i.e. by its filling inter- and intracellular spaces of the dead corneocytes, and to some extent perhaps at the molecular level by binding to cell protein macromolecules, both keratinous and non-keratinous. The aggregate result, however, is to provide an aqueous lubricating system for the cellular lattice structure of the stratum corneum, a lubrication that accounts for unusual pliability of the stratum corneum.

Facilitating this aqueous lubricating system, but not substituting for it, are lipid materials, normally formed by the epidermis and the sebaceous glands or ones which may be therapeutically applied externally, that act principally to restrain evaporative loss of water. This role of lipids can be illustrated by simple experiments with desiccated isolated strips of plantar calluses, which are decidedly hard and brittle. Such strips soaked in anhydrous oils or greases remain hard and brittle. Soaked in water, they become decidedly soft and supple, and if then covered with an occlusive oil or grease remain so for prolonged periods. This illustration, devised by one of us a quarter century ago as a teaching device to display the findings of Blank, probably is not adequate to explain completely the role of physiologic lipids found in normal stratum corneum and which may play roles somewhat more complex but which must, in the end, serve to enhance stratum corneum hydration.

Keratolysis

Hydrating agents, affecting the physical properties of the stratum corneum without otherwise altering structural integrity, are to be distinguished from those agents that should be properly known as keratolytics. Keratolytics are in fact protein denaturants which have the capability of disintegrating the stratum corneum to one degree or another, to solubilize one or more fractions which normally are insoluble. While some investigational use has been made of agents in this category, they have found little clinical application for the reason, one may suppose, that their denaturing effects extend beyond the stratum corneum to cause what is generically known as irritation. Some agents have found wide use, however, as ingredients of hair waving procedures, particularly thiol reducing agents.

Distinct from hydrating agents and keratolytics that affect the stratum corneum directly are agents we categorize as keratinization modifiers. In recent publications[3] we have reported that α-hydroxy acids as a class, and some β-

hydroxy acids, consistently normalize the stratum corneum in the several types of ichthyosis after several days topical application, as well as exerting substantial similar effects in several other disorders. This and further work lead us to reach certain conclusions on what the normal controls of keratinization might be. A short review of some of these studies is provided below.

α-Hydroxy acids in therapy of dry skin, ichthyosis and other disorders

All compounds that we have studied for effects on keratinization have been initially evaluated on a series of over twenty patients with ichthyosis of several types. Many of the compounds have been evaluated for therapeutic effects on larger series of patients with dry skin; several have been used therapeutically for comedonous acne; and a few have been used in therapy of a diverse group of disorders including palmar and plantar hyperkeratosis, Darier's disease, lichen simplex chronicus and others. Reduction in stratum corneum accumulation has been readily demonstrable in all disorders in response to two–four times daily topical application of the compounds formulated as 5–20% oil-in-water creams, as solutions and as gels.

Table 1.2 Compounds known to promote normal keratinization in ichthyosis

Citric acid	Mandelic acid
Glycolic acid	Mucic acid
Glucuronic acid	Pyruvic acid
Galacturonic acid	Methyl pyruvate
Glucuronolactone	Ethyl pyruvate
Gluconolactone	β-Phenyllactic acid
α-Hydroxybutyric acid	β-Phenylpyruvic acid
α-Hydroxyisobutyric acid	Saccharic acid
Lactic acid	Tartaric acid
Atrolactic acid	Tartronic acid
Malic acid	β-Hydroxybutyric acid

Twenty-two compounds (Table 1.2) incorporated into hydrophilic ointment USP have been found to restore toward normal the hyperkeratotic skin of the ichthyoses as evaluated clinically and histologically. Of this group seventeen are α-hydroxy acids, four are α-keto acids or esters thereof, and in one the hydroxyl group is in the β position.

The sequence of histologic and clinical changes in lamellar ichthyosis[3] suggests that the effect of these compounds on the skin are mediated by means of their influence at the level of the underlying epidermis insofar as after several days of topical treatment a normal skin surface abruptly appears clinically, consequent to sheet-like desquamation of the entire thickened stratum corneum. This is correlated histologically with the emergence of a normally thin stratum corneum and reduction in thickness of the epidermis. No clinical or histologic evidence of dissolution of stratum corneum is found, nor have we been able to demonstrate any evidence of solubilization of stratum corneum by these compounds in *in vitro* experiments (unpublished). We conclude, therefore, that the effects seen are due to influences on the epidermal keratinization process.

Hydroxy-keto acids in keratinization control

All integumental epithelial cells of the epidermis, skin appendages, oral cavity and conjunctiva, as well as epithelial cells in other locations such as in the bronchial tree and genital tract, have the capability of pronounced keratinization under suitable conditions. This suggests that keratinization may be a primitive attribute of these cells and that expression of other differentiated functions requires simultaneous suppression or modulation of keratinization. It seems possible that α-hydroxy or keto-acids or immediately related compounds carry out such suppression or modulation. The specificity of molecular attributes associated with suppression of keratinization may be at least partially discernible from information now available.

From our studies on ichthyosis we conclude that the carboxyl group is indispensable for keratinization control. It has not yet been possible though to determine whether a hydroxy or keto group is required at the α position insofar as these groups are readily interconvertible under physiologic conditions. The fact that pyruvic acid is more effective than lactic acid in topical therapy of epidermolytic hyperkeratosis[3] and in the ichthyotic disease called spiny hyperkeratosis suggests that the keto form may provide heightened activity.

The length and configuration of the remainder of the molecule also clearly modifies the activity, although requirements of this are not clear as yet. Increasing lengths of side chain are, in general, correlated with decreasing activity; α-hydroxylauric acid, for example, is found to be totally ineffective as topical treatment of lamellar ichthyosis. The side chain is not required to be a straight chain since one of the more active compounds has been phenyl glycolic (mandelic) acid.

Hydroxylation at the β position can confer a degree of activity. Having partial activity, for example, are β-hydroxy butyric and salicylic (o-hydroxybenzoic) acids. However, these are distinctly less active than the α-hydroxy acids.

These findings now provide a basis for formulating a hypothesis on the defect accounting for the ichthyotic skin in Refsum's disease. Deficient activity of an α-hydroxylating enzyme of phytanic acid has been reported to exist in this disease[4,5]. While it was postulated that defective fatty acid metabolism may itself account for the ichthyotic skin changes, we would at this time postulate that the deficiency of α-hydroxylation may be more general and account for decreased amounts of other α-hydroxy acids that normally function to modulate keratinization.

Active forms of vitamin A

The role of α-hydroxy or keto acids may also be evident as far as vitamin A and its modulative suppression of keratinization are concerned. It seems relevant that the acid form of the vitamin, while inactive in promoting normal vision and reproduction, can completely promote normal differentiation and reverse the epithelial hyperkeratinization found in vitamin A deficiency[6,7]. Our own studies on agents that reverse the extreme hyperkeratinization found in the skin of the rhino mouse, some results of which have been published[8], and our studies on follicular hyperkeratinization in acne indicate that vitamin A acid is most effective in normalizing epidermal keratinization, with vitamin A aldehyde next most effective. There is reason to believe, however, that one or more metabolites of vitamin A acid may have greater specific activity. Some such metabolites have been identified, and have been found to contain one hydroxy group in the molecule[9]. The role of vitamin A compounds in restraining keratinization is quite comprehensive, extending beyond that of the α-hydroxy or keto acids, for in vitamin A deficiency hyperkeratinization is not limited to the skin but is pronounced in other epithelial tissues as well, such as that of the eye and uterus[10]. The recent therapeutic trials of Peck (see Chapter 23) with the cis-isomer of vitamin A acid showing that oral administration of this compound can exert beneficial effects on cases of ichthyosis, suggest that vitamin A acid (possibly hydroxylated) and groups of α-hydroxy or keto acids may interdigitate as regulators of keratinization.

PROJECTIONS

The advances in what at this time seem to represent improved understanding of the ichthyoses have been made by means of studying the response of these diseases in patients seeking help for their affliction. While topical therapy with α-hydroxy or keto acids has been effective and safe for these patients, patient non-compliance with the requirement of continuous twice-daily whole-body applications of greasy topical formulations, points to the need for safe systemic therapy. Several of our patients have been fed several grams daily of lactic acid. No objectively discernible improvement has occurred, but neither has there been any detectable elevation of serum lactate or pyruvate. Such results were anticipated for it is to be expected that these substances are promptly metabolized in their first pass through the liver. We have since initiated trial therapy in one patient with oral mandelic acid, a non-degradable α-hydroxy acid used for many years in large dosage as a urinary antiseptic. Our preliminary observations suggest that distinct improvement may be achievable by such therapy. There is need for further clinical investigations and pharmacologic explorations, however.

Several clues now are present on the possible nature of the ichthyoses and on potential categories of agents for treatment. Needed are studies to determine whether biochemical defects in structural keratinous proteins exist; whether the thickened stratum corneum is due to too great a cellular cohesiveness, and if so whether this is related to abnormal inter-cellular adhesive materials, e.g. mucopolysaccharides; whether the thickened stratum corneum is less hygroscopic than normal, and if so what might be the missing humectant.

It is unclear whether the agents now known to be beneficial in diseases of disturbed keratinization exert their effects at the level of DNA, RNA, the messenger systems between them and final synthetic pathways, or other metabolic systems that may be conceptualized. It should be emphasized, however, that while all the ichthyotic disorders have genetic determinants, presumably residing in DNA, the manifest defects are likely post-transcriptional and can be ameliorated or altered by pharmacological means.

References

1. Blank, I. H. (1952). Factors which influence the water content of the stratum corneum. *J. Invest. Dermatol.*, **18**, 433
2. Blank, I. H. (1953). Further observations on factors which influence the water content of the stratum corneum. *J. Invest. Dermatol.*, **21**, 259
3. Van Scott, E. J. and Yu, R. J. (1974). Control of keratinization with α-hydroxy acids and related compounds. I. Topical treatment of ichthyotic disorders. *Arch. Dermatol.*, **110**, 586
4. Herndon, J. H., Jr., Steinberg, D., Uhlendorf, B. W. and Fales, H. M. (1969). Refsum's disease: Characterization of the enzyme defect in cell culture. *J. Clin. Invest.*, **48**, 1017
5. Mize, C. E., Herndon, J. H., Jr., Blass, J. P., Milne, G. W. A., Follansbee, C., Laudat, P. and Steinberg, D. (1969). Localization of the oxidative defect in phytanic acid degradation in patients with Refsum's disease. *J. Clin. Invest.*, **48**, 1033
6. Arens, J. F. and Van Dorp, D. A. (1946). Synthesis of some compounds possessing vitamin A activity. *Nature (London)*, **157**, 190
7. Dowling J. E. and Wald, G. (1960). The biological function of vitamin A acid. *Proc. Nat. Acad. Sci., USA*, **46**, 587
8. Van Scott, E. J. (1972). Experimental animal integumental models for screening potential dermatologic drugs. In: W. Montagna, E. J. Van Scott and R. B. Stoughton (eds.), *Pharmacology and the Skin*, p. 523. (New York: Appleton-Century-Crofts)
9. Yagishita, K., Sundaresan, P. R. and Wolf G. (1964). A biologically active vitamin A metabolite. *Federation Proc., Fed. Am. Soc. Exp. Biol.*, **23**, 294
10. Moore, T. (1967). Effects of vitamin A deficiency in animals. In: W. H. Sebrell, Jr. and R. S. Harris (eds.), *The Vitamins*, 2nd Ed., Vol. I, p. 245. (New York and London: Academic Press)

2
Essential Fatty Acids and Skin Scaliness

C. PROTTEY

The essential fatty acids (EFA) are long-chain unsaturated lipids so named as they are essential to the diet of mammals and cannot be synthesized *de novo*, as are all other lipids. There are two major EFAs[1], both of ω-6 configuration (denoting the position of the first methylene-interrupted double bond, numbered from the methyl end of the chain) and their structures are shown in Figure 2.1. Linoleic acid is the most common EFA, and arachidonic acid is a chain elongation product of it.

Figure 2.1 ω-6 fatty acids

$$CH_3-CH_2-Cn_2\cdot CH_2\cdot CH_2-CH=CH-CH_2-CH=CH-CH_2-CH_2-CH_2-CH_2-$$
18   13   12   10   9

$$CH_2-CH_2\cdot CH_2 \qquad n$$

Linoleic or ω-6 octadecadienoic acid

$$CH_3-CH_2-CH_2-CH_2-CH_2-CH=CH-CH_2-CH=CH-CH_2-CH=CH-CH_2-CH=CH-$$
15   14   12   11   9   8   6   5

$$CH_2-CH_2-CH_2-COOH$$
1

Arachidonic or ω-6 eicosatetraenoic acid

When mammals are deprived of EFA in the diet 'EFA-deficiency' results, with characteristic abnormalities, particularly in the skin[1]. The albino rat has received most study, and Table 2.1 lists changes that occur in the skin. In this paper two features are discussed more fully, namely scaliness and 'leakiness',

Table 2.1   Abnormalities of the skin in EFA-deficient rats

1. Coarse fur, clogged with dandruff-like flakes
2. Scaly paws and tail
3. No brown 'Sebum' on skin surface
4. Hyperplastic epidermis, increased mitosis
5. Dense compacted stratum corneum
6. Reduced inflammatory response
7. Impaired prostaglandin synthesis
8. Abnormal sterol esterification
9. Impaired barrier function — skin more permeable to water
10. Reduced amounts of ω-6 acids in skin phospholipids
11. Accumulation of ω-9 acid

and I shall attempt to assign specific functions of EFAs in the restoration of these features to normal.

The feet of rats raised from weaning on EFA-deficient diet are scaly and cracked and this occurs generally within 2 weeks. The tail also exhibits scaliness and 'ringing', and later, necrosis of the tip. Microscopically the dorsal epidermis is thickened and hyperplastic, with a greater than normal number of cells in mitosis, an elaborated stratum granulosum, increased keratohyalin, and a highly compacted stratum corneum[1].

Much of what is known about skin scaliness in EFA-deficiency originates from the work of Basnayake and Sinclair[2], who found that when rats were given EFA-deficient diets they grew at reduced rates, within a few weeks scaliness of the feet and tail developed, and transepidermal water loss (TEWL) rose by a factor of 10. When EFA was reintroduced to the diet the abnormalities disappeared, that is, the condition was reversible. We have shown[3] that skin abnormalities of the EFA-deficient rat may be reversed also by topical application of linoleic acid, and this is as effective as feeding. Within five days of rubbing sunflower seed oil (a rich source of linoleic acid) onto the dorsal skin of deficient rats, TEWL was restored to normal, more rapidly than the scaliness was healed.

There are two possible mechanisms by which impaired barrier function (i.e. high TEWL) may be restored by topical linoleic acid, namely, by direct involvement of linoleic acid in the skin membranes responsible for maintaining the permeability barrier, or, after conversion to prostaglandins, by controlling the replicative property of the epidermis and the process of keratinization, both of which are disrupted in EFA-deficiency. Linoleic acid, derived from the diet, can be further desaturated to γ-linolenic acid and then elongated to dihomo-γ-linolenic acid, a precursor of PGE_1, and $PGF_{1\alpha}$. Dihomo-γ-linolenic acid may then be further desaturated to arachidonic acid, the precursor of PGE_2 and $PGF_{2\alpha}$[1]. Could it be that when linoleic acid is rubbed onto the skin, some is converted to prostaglandins and thereby regulates disrupted keratinization, consequently restoring impaired barrier function and scaliness to normal? Figure 2.2 shows that when various ω-6 acids were tested[4], only linoleic acid and its desaturation product γ-linolenic acid restored TEWL to normal when

12

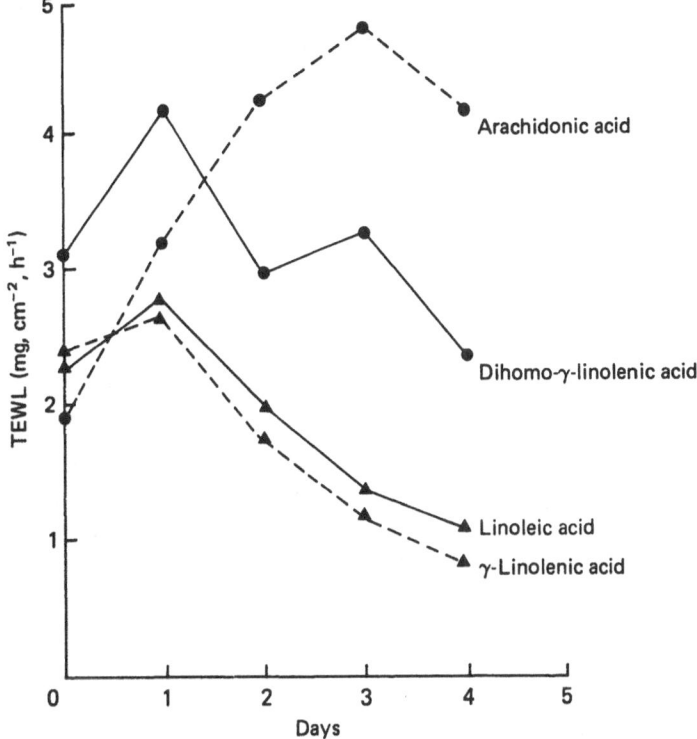

Figure 2.2 Effect of topical action of ω-6 acids on TEWL

applied topically. Table 2.2 shows that PGE$_1$ and PGE$_2$ applied as butyl esters had no effect[5]. None influenced skin scaliness during the course of application, although Ziboh and Hsia[6] reported that PGE$_2$ rubbed onto the scaly feet of EFA-deficient rats, healed the skin. Following application of the various fatty acids, all were incorporated into epidermal lecithin, the two that were incorporated the most, linoleic and γ-linolenic acids, being those that lowered TEWL (Table 2.3). We never observed conversion of any applied fatty acids to arachidonic acid, suggesting that this strain of rat is incapable of performing this reaction. We have recently found[5] that linoleic acid exerts this restorative effect upon TEWL even when prostaglandin synthesis is blocked by

Table 2.2 Butyl prostaglandins and TEWL in EFA-deficient rats

Treatment	TEWL (mg cm^{-2} h^{-1}) at increasing treatment periods					
	0	Day 1	Day 2	Day 3	Day 4	Day 5
Controls	2.3	2.3	1.7	1.8	1.7	2.3
Butyl PGE$_1$	2.2	2.3	2.1	2.4	2.3	2.5
Butyl PGE$_2$	2.3	2.0	1.6	2.0	2.0	1.7

Table 2.3   Fatty acid incorporation after topical application to EFA deficient rats

Chain length of fatty acid applied	Percentage of applied fatty acid incorporated into epidermal lecithin	
	Untreated	*After treatment*
18:2	1.6	10.9
γ18:3	0.2	5.5
20:3	trace	1.0
20:4	1.8	2.8

indomethacin. Thus, linoleic and γ-linolenic acids are the only two EFA's that restore barrier function to normal in EFA-deficiency. This restoration does not involve either arachidonic acid or prostaglandins.

Regarding skin scaliness and EFA-deficiency, others[7] had shown that arachidonic acid, not linoleic acid, was more important (i.e. the opposite to skin permeability).This was confirmed[5] by giving rats either linoleic or arachidonic acid by intraperitoneal injection. This approach was chosen rather than topical application as arachidonic acid is synthesized in the liver, so any of this lipid reaching the skin after linoleic acid administration must be transported there from the liver via the blood. Figure 2.3 shows that linoleic

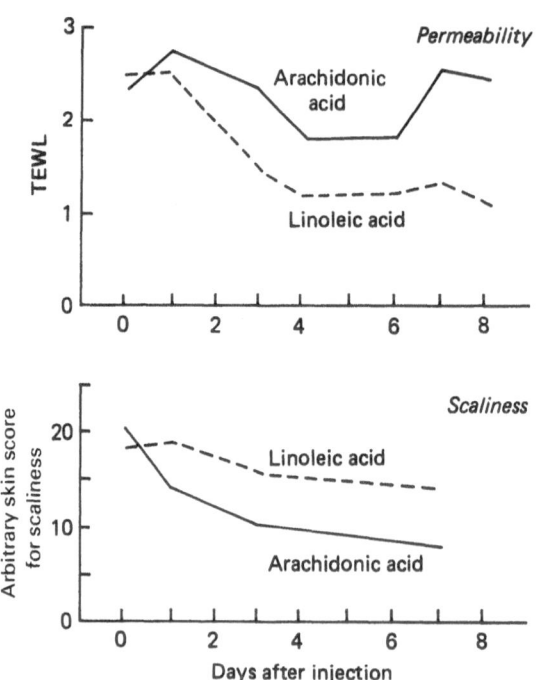

Figure 2.3   Effect of linoleic and arachidonic acids by I.P. injection on skin permeability and scaliness

acid was more effective than arachidonic acid in the repair of TEWL—con-
firming our earlier findings[4] with topical application. With the healing of
scaliness, however, arachidonic acid was more effective than linoleic acid.

It was thought that this specific function of arachidonic acid, quite separable
from that of linoleic acid, involves conversion to prostaglandins. This was
supported by studies on the hypophysectomized rat. Now the hypophysectomized rat bears striking similarities to the EFA-deficient rat[8] (growth

Table 2.4 Skin permeability (TEWL) in hypophysectomized (hypox)
rats

Animals	TEWL (mg, cm^{-2}, h^{-1})
Normals (10)	0.370 ± 0.190
Hypox, 8 weeks (3)	0.309 ± 0.154
Hypox, 15 weeks (3)	0.270 ± 0.049
EFA-deficient, 12 weeks (42)	2.313 ± 0.379

is impaired, the fur is coarse, tail and paw skin are scaly and cracked). Yet the
hypophysectomized rat is not EFA-deficient. Skin permeability data are given
in Table 2.4, and are quite normal, unlike EFA-deficient rat skin. Lipid analyses
(Table 2.5) showed that unlike EFA-deficient rat skin, hypophysectomized rats

Table 2.5 Fatty acid content (percentage) hypophysectomized (hypox)
EFA-deficient and normal (control) rats

Chain length of fatty acids	Animals		
	Normal	hypox	EFA-deficient
16:0	25.1	18.0	19.3
18:0	15.0	17.2	9.6
18:1	17.2	18.2	29.6
18:2	15.4	22.3	1.6
20:3 ω-9	0	2.7	8.6
20:4 ω-6	3.4	9.9	1.8

contain more linoleic acid than normal. As scaliness of these animals was
observed, this confirmed that skin scaliness and impaired barrier function are
separable phenomena.

Although hypophysectomized rats contain more arachidonic acid than
normal, ω-9 eicosatrienoic acid is also found. Prostaglandin formation in the
EFA-deficient rat is severely impaired, and ω-9 eicosatrienoic acid is a potent
inhibitor[9]. This suggested that in the hypophysectomized rat similarly,
prostaglandin synthesis was inhibited. Total body prostaglandin synthesis was
monitored by measuring excretion of prostaglandin metabolites in the urine[5]
(Table 2.6). In the rat derivatives of tetranorprostane dioic acid are found in

Table 2.6   Urinary prostaglandin metabolites* in the rat

	Per animal per day (μg)
Normal rats	16.7
EFA-deficient rats	4.03
Hypox rats	1.24

* Determined as tetranorprostanedioic acid.

the urine and are derived from endogenous prostaglandins. The daily output of metabolites was 16.7 μg tetranorprostane dioate for normal rats, 4.03 μg for EFA-deficient rats, and 1.24 μg for hypophysectomized rats. This confirmed that hypophysectomized rats, like EFA-deficient rats, cannot synthesize adequate prostaglandins.

It is not proved that in the skin of hypophysectomized rats prostaglandin synthesis is prevented, neither is it proved that this is the cause of scaliness, but the above data support these ideas. It is thus suggested that the function of arachidonic acid in the skin is to serve as precursor to prostaglandins, which, in turn, participate in the regulation of epidermal turnover, and, indirectly, skin scaliness. When prostaglandin synthesis in the skin is prevented, as in either EFA-deficiency or after hypophysectomy, skin scaliness results.

Functions and significance of the essential fatty acids, linoleic acid and arachidonic acid are summarized in Table 2.7

Table 2.7 Functions and significance of EFA in skin

Linoleic acid
1. Not synthesized by mammals, but required in the diet
2. Transported to the skin via the blood
3. Incorporated in skin structural lipids of membranes and enzymes
4. Important in barrier properties (permeability, percutaneous absorption)
5. Absence from skin causes faulty barrier properties of stratum corneum

Arachidonic acid
1. Not synthesized in skin (but in liver from dietary linoleic acid)
2. Transported to the skin via the blood
3. Incorporated in skin phospholipids (lecithin, phosphatidylethanolamine)
4. Precursor of prostaglandins which:
    (a) regulate epidermal homeostasis
    (b) mediate inflammation
5. Absence from skin influences regulation of keratinization and inflammation

References

1. Prottey, C. (1976). Essential fatty acids and the skin. *Br. J. Dermatol.*, **94,** 579
2. Basnayake, V. and Sinclair, H. M. (1956). The effect of deficiency of essential fatty acids upon the skin. In: G. Popjak and E. LeBreton (eds), *Biochemical Problems of Lipids*, p. 476. (London: Butterworth)

3. Prottey, C., Hartop, P. J., Black, J. G. and McCormack, J. I. (1976). The repair of impaired epidermal barrier function in rats by the cutaneous application of linoleic acid. *Br. J. Dermatol.*, **94,** 13

4. Hartop, P. J. and Prottey, C. (1976). Changes in transepidermal water loss and the composition of epidermal lecithin after applications of pure fatty and triglycerides to the skin of essential fatty acid-deficient rats. *Br. J. Dermatol.*, **95,** 225

5. Prottey, C. (1977). Investigations of functions of essential fatty acids. *Br. J. Dermatol.*, **97,** 29

6. Ziboh, V. A. and Hsia, S. L. (1972). Effects of prostaglandin E_2 on rat skin: inhibition of sterol ester biosynthesis and clearing of scaly lesions in essential fatty acid deficiency. *J. Lipid Res.*, **13,** 458

7. Holman, R. T. (1970). Biological activities of and requirements for polyunsaturated acids. In: R. T. Homan (ed), *Progress in the Chemistry of Fats and Other Lipids*. Vol. IX, pt. 5, p. 611. (Oxford: Pergamon)

8. Haeffner, E. W. and Privett, D. S. (1973). Development of dermal symptoms resembling those of an essential fatty acid deficiency in immature hypophysectomized rats. *J. Nutr.*, **103,** 74

9. Ziboh, V. A., Vanderhoek, J. Y. and Lands, W. E. M. (1974). Inhibition of sheep vesicular gland oxygenase by unsaturated fatty acids from the skin of essential fatty acid deficient rats. *Prostaglandins*, **5,** 233

3
Epidermal Lipogenesis in Ichthyosis

MARY F. COOPER, D. McGIBBON and S. SHUSTER

INTRODUCTION

Several lines of evidence point to a connection between lipid metabolism and scaly skin. Inhibitors of cholesterol biosynthesis such as triparanol and nicotinic acid can produce scaly lesions superficially resembling ichthyosis[1]. A disturbance of cutaneous sterol ester biosynthesis accompanies the hyperkeratosis of essential fatty acid deficiency[2], and increased ratios of free sterol to sterol esters have been reported in psoriasis[3,4] and atopic eczema[5]. We have recently shown[6] that epidermal lipid biosynthesis is increased in lesions of psoriasis and lichen simplex, with the free sterol fraction affected more than other lipid classes.

Epidermal sterol biosynthesis in ichthyosis vulgaris was studied by Summerly and Yardley[7], who found that acetate incorporation into sterols was increased (but not significantly so). These results were weight-corrected, and so may have been distorted by the presence of inert scale in the ichthyotic samples. We therefore decided to reinvestigate sterol biosynthesis in ichthyosis, within the context of total epidermal lipogenesis.

Methods

The subjects for this study were as shown in Table 3.1. The control group consisted of nine males and two females, aged from 41 to 73 and with a variety of minor skin disorders not involving hyperkeratinization.

For measurement of lipogenesis, two 4 mm punch biopsies of untreated skin

Table 3.1 Epidermal lipogenesis from [^{14}C]glucose in ichthyosis vulgaris

Subject	Age and sex	Type of ichthyosis	^{14}C incorporation into lipids (d.p.m./biopsy)
1	60♀	Autosomal dominant	7 580
2	61♀	Autosomal dominant	8 330
3	63♂*	Autosomal dominant*	3 050
4	68♀	Autosomal dominant	10 730
5	39♂	Sex-linked recessive	8 400
6	67♂	Sex-linked recessive	7 260
7	59♂	Acquired	7 900
	Control group (mean $\pm$ SEM, $n = 11$)		4 540 $\pm$ 430

* No evidence of hyperkeratosis in adjacent skin.

were taken with lignocaine anaesthesia from the shoulder blade region of the back. A third biopsy of adjacent skin was taken for routine histology. All but one of the ichthyotic group (subject number 3) showed evidence of hyperkeratosis at this body site.

The method of measuring lipogenesis has been reported in detail elsewhere[6]. Briefly, intact skin biopsies were incubated for three hours at 37 °C in Krebs Ringer bicarbonate buffer, gassed with $O_2 + 5\%$ CO_2 and containing antibiotics and 2 mM [U-^{14}C]glucose (5 mCi/mmol). After incubation the skin was treated with 0.5% acetic acid to loosen the epidermis, which could then be peeled away as an intact disc. Total lipids were extracted and separated into classes by thin layer chromatography on silicic acid, and the radioactivity in each spot was measured by scintillation counting.

Results and discussion

The ^{14}C incorporation into total epidermal lipids is shown in Table 3.1 and Figure 3.1. In those ichthyotic subjects who showed histological evidence of hyperkeratosis on the back, ^{14}C incorporation was significantly higher than in controls ($P < 0.001$). However, in the single subject who showed no histological evidence of hyperkeratosis, lipogenic activity was within the normal range (Table 3.1).

The reason for the observed increase in lipid labelling is not immediately obvious. None of the biopsies taken for histology showed evidence of epidermal thickening, and so the results cannot be explained in terms of an increased mass of viable tissue per unit area of epidermis. The use of a labelled precursor in substrate, rather than tracer, quantities, makes it unlikely that the finding is an artifact caused by changes in metabolic pool sizes. Nor does it seem possible to account for the results in terms of increased cell turnover, as the rate of epidermal proliferation in both autosomal dominant and sex-linked recessive ichthyosis is within normal limits[8]. Whether lipid turnover is

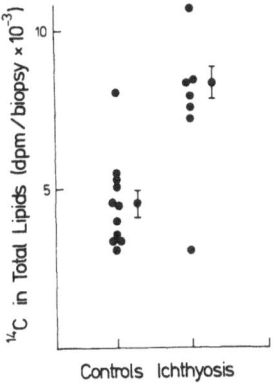

Figure 3.1 ^{14}C incorporation into total epidermal lipids of punch biopsies from control and ichthyotic subjects. Mean $\pm$ SEM are shown for the control group, and for the six ichthyotic subjects who showed histological evidence of hyperkeratosis in adjacent skin

increased independently of cell turnover, or whether there is a net increase in lipid biosynthesis per cell, are questions which will require further study.

The pattern of lipid labelling (Table 3.2) showed no significant differences between the control and ichthyotic groups, except for small increases in the

Table 3.2 Distribution of ^{14}C between lipid classes in control and ichthyotic epidermis

Lipid class	% of total lipid labelling (mean $\pm$ SEM)	
	Control (n = 11)	Ichthyosis (n = 7)
Polar lipids	60.3 $\pm$ 1.3	54.6 $\pm$ 3.6
Free sterols	6.9 $\pm$ 0.8	5.8 $\pm$ 0.8
Free fatty acids	5.7 $\pm$ 0.6	8.6 $\pm$ 1.2‡
Monoglycerides	3.9 $\pm$ 0.3	4.1 $\pm$ 0.3
1,2-diglycerides	5.8 $\pm$ 0.4	8.6 $\pm$ 0.5§
1,3-diglycerides*	3.0 $\pm$ 0.4	3.2 $\pm$ 0.6
Triglycerides†	9.0 $\pm$ 0.9	11.2 $\pm$ 2.0
Wax esters + sterol esters	1.4 $\pm$ 0.2	0.7 $\pm$ 0.3
Squalene	1.4 $\pm$ 0.3	1.7 $\pm$ 0.6

* May also contain fatty alcohols.
† May also contain glyceryl ether lipids.
‡ $p < 0.05$.
§ $p < 0.001$.

relative labelling of the free fatty acid and 1,2-diglyceride fractions in ichthyosis. This may perhaps indicate that the further steps in lipid biosynthesis from these precursors have become rate-limiting; alternatively, an increase in lipid turnover might produce the same result. No increase was seen in the relative labelling of free sterols; this is in contrast with our previous findings in psoriasis and lichen simplex[6], and suggests that a specific alteration in sterol metabolism is not a necessary accompaniment of hyperkeratosis.

The present findings add further to the evidence of a disturbance in lipid metabolism in a variety of scaly disorders. The precise definition of these disturbances, and whether they are cause or effect, will require further study.

Acknowledgements

We wish to thank Mrs. Jennifer Alcock for expert technical assistance. This work was supported by grants from the Wellcome Trust and the Medical Research Council.

References

1. Yardley, H. J. (1969). Sterols and keratinisation. *Br. J. Dermatol.*, **81** (Suppl. 2), 29
2. Ziboh, V. A. and Hsia, S. L. (1972). Effects of prostaglandin E_2 on rat skin: inhibition of sterol ester biosynthesis and clearing of scaly lesions in essential fatty acid deficiency. *J. Lipid Res.*, **13,** 458
3. von Glasenapp, I. and Leonhardi, G. (1953). Uber den Cholesterinstoffwechsel in der Gesunden und der psoriatisch veranderten Haut. *Arch. Dermatol. Syphilol.*, **96,** 148
4. Wheatley, V. R. and Farber, E. M. (1961). Studies on the chemical composition of psoriatic scales. *J. Invest. Dermatol.*, **36,** 199
5. Mustakallio, K. K., Kiistala, U., Piha, H. J. and Nieminen, E. (1967). Epidermal lipids in Besnier's Prurigo (atopic eczema). *Ann. Med. Exp. Biol. Fenn.*, **45,** 323
6. Cooper, M. F., McGrath, H. and Shuster, S. (1976). Epidermal lipid metabolism in psoriasis and lichen simplex. *Br. J. Dermatol.*, **94,** 369
7. Summerly, R. and Yardley, H. J. (1967). Cholesterol synthesis in ichthyosis vulgaris. *Br. J. Dermatol.*, **79,** 378
8. Frost, P. and Weinstein, G. D. (1971). Ichthyosiform dermatoses. In: T. B. Fitzpatrick *et al.* (ed.) *Dermatology in General Medicine*, pp. 249–265. (New York: McGraw-Hill)

4
Lipid Synthesis in Ichthyotic Conditions

P. J. DYKES and R. MARKS

INTRODUCTION

The association of abnormal lipid metabolism with disordered keratinization has been apparent for some time. Drugs such as Triparanol[1] and nicotinic acid[2] which influence cholesterol metabolism have been responsible for a dry scaly skin condition resembling autosomal dominant ichthyosis (ADI). Similar rashes are seen in both essential fatty acid deficient animals[3] and humans[4]. Refsum's disease (Heredopathia Atactica Polyneuritiformis) has also been reported as having an ichthyotic component[5]. In this disease there is an accumulation of phytanic acid in the tissues together with an apparent substitution of this fatty acid for linoleic and arachidonic acid in the phospholipid moieties[6,7].

That lipid compositional changes occur during keratinization is also beyond dispute. Both Long[8] and more recently Gray and Yardley[9] have demonstrated altered lipid composition as a function of depth in the epidermis. Such changes are probably associated with the degeneration of the nuclear membrane and the cytoplasmic organelles. Summerly and Yardley[10] measured the rate of biosynthesis of total sterols in ADI and found an increased biosynthesis of sterol per mg tissue when compared to normals. Although this increase was not statistically significant, the presence of scale may have biased the results unfavourably.

We have investigated the *in vitro* rate of [14C]acetate incorporation in ADI and compared this with normal values and a patient with Refsum's disease. The *in vitro* incorporation of other radioactive precursors was also studied in the ADI patients.

23

MATERIALS AND METHODS

Patients

Seven patients with autosomal dominant ichthyosis (four males, three females, age range 26–70 years) were compared with six normal volunteers (four males, two females, age range 25–64 years) and a patient with an ichthyotic eruption associated with Refsum's disease. The patient with Refsum's disease is described in detail elsewhere (see Chapter 8).

Skin sampling and culture

Appendage free epidermis was obtained from the thighs of individuals using a Castroviejo keratotome set at 0.4 mm. Specimens of skin thus obtained were cut into 50 mm squares and incubated *in vitro* with radioactively labelled thymidine, proline, histidine and acetate.

In vitro incorporation of ^{14}C acetate

Incubation of skin specimens — Specimens were incubated at 37 °C in Eagles MEM containing 10% human serum and 25 μCi/ml of ^{14}C labelled acetate (1-^{14}C acetic acid, sodium salt, specific activity = 60 mCi/mmole, The Radiochemical Centre, Amersham). After 4 hours incubation, the skin samples were rinsed briefly in saline and stored at −20 °C until analysed by thin layer chromatography (TLC).

Lipid extraction and analysis — Skin specimens were homogenized in distilled water and precipitated with 10% perchloric acid. The precipitates were washed with 2% perchloric acid and distilled water and then extracted twice with chloroform–methanol (2:1 v/v). Extracts were pooled and analysed by chromatography on precoated thin layer plates (20 × 20 cm) of silica gel 60 (Merck, A.G. Darmstadt, Germany) after activation at 110 °C for 30 minutes. Lipid analysis was performed as described by Summerly and Woodbury[11]. Plates were developed firstly in hexane–benzene (1:1, v/v) and secondly in the same dimension with petroleum ether (b.p. 60–80 °C)–diethyl ether–acetic acid (80:20:1, by vol).

Phospholipids were analysed using the single development system of chloroform–methanol–acetic acid–water (50:30:8:4, v/v), described by Skipski, Peterson and Barclay[12].

After development the radioactive bands were located using a Panax thin layer scanner and provisionally identified by co-chromatography with reference compounds. Those areas corresponding to the bands were then removed from the plate and the radioactivity eluted and estimated by scintillation counting. Results are expressed as d.p.m. per sq.mm per hour.

In vitro incorporation of ^3H thymidine, proline and histidine

Specimens were incubated at 37 °C in Eagles MEM containing 1 μCi/ml of either tritiated thymidine or proline or histidine and processed for scintillation counting as previously described[13,14]. Results are expressed as d.p.m. per sq.mm per hour.

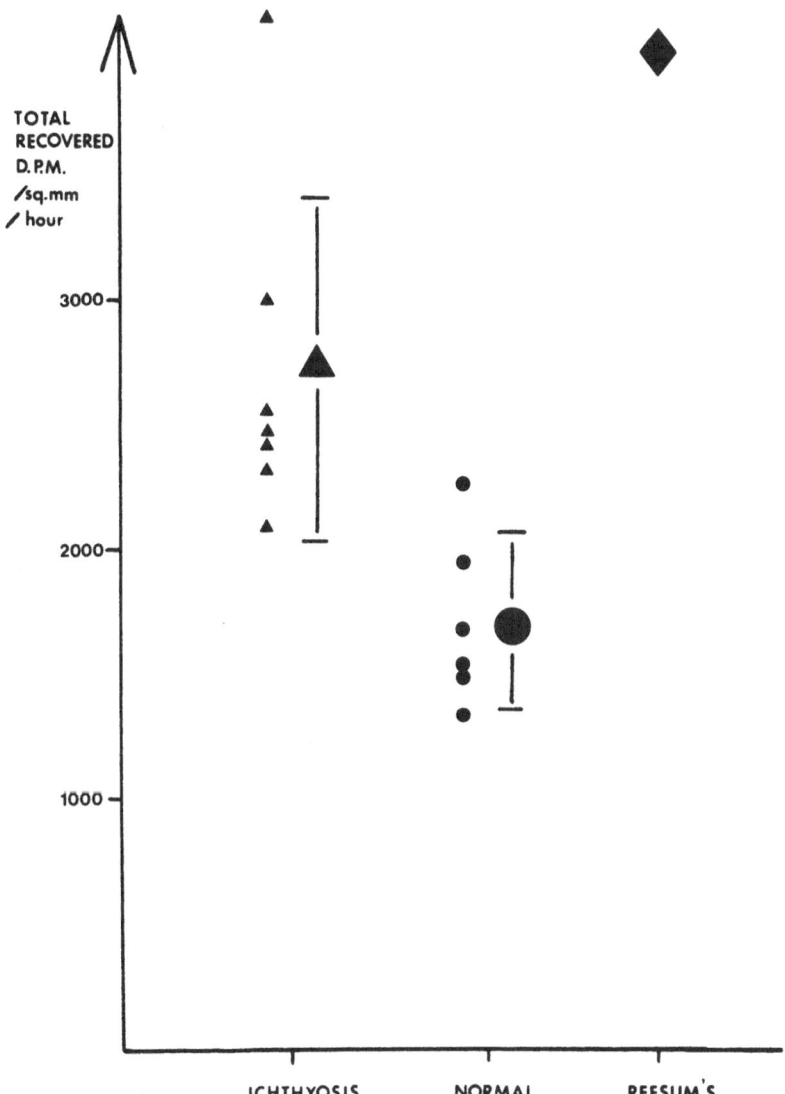

Figure 4.1 Total d.p.m. per square mm per hour recovered from TLC plates after analysis of ^{14}C acetate labelled lipids extracted from normal and ichthyotic epidermis. Each value shown is the mean value of two skin specimens analysed. The mean ± standard deviation of both groups is also given. The value obtained in the Refsum's patient is shown

RESULTS

Incorporation of ¹⁴C acetate into total recoverable lipids

The total radioactivity recoverable from the TLC plates for both groups and the patient with Refsum's disease is compared in Figure 4.1. A quantitative difference is apparent, there being approximately 60% more radioactivity recoverable in the ichthyosis group than in the normals. This difference was significant ($P < 0.01$) according to the Student 't' test. In the patient with Refsum's disease an increase of 130% compared to normal was noted.

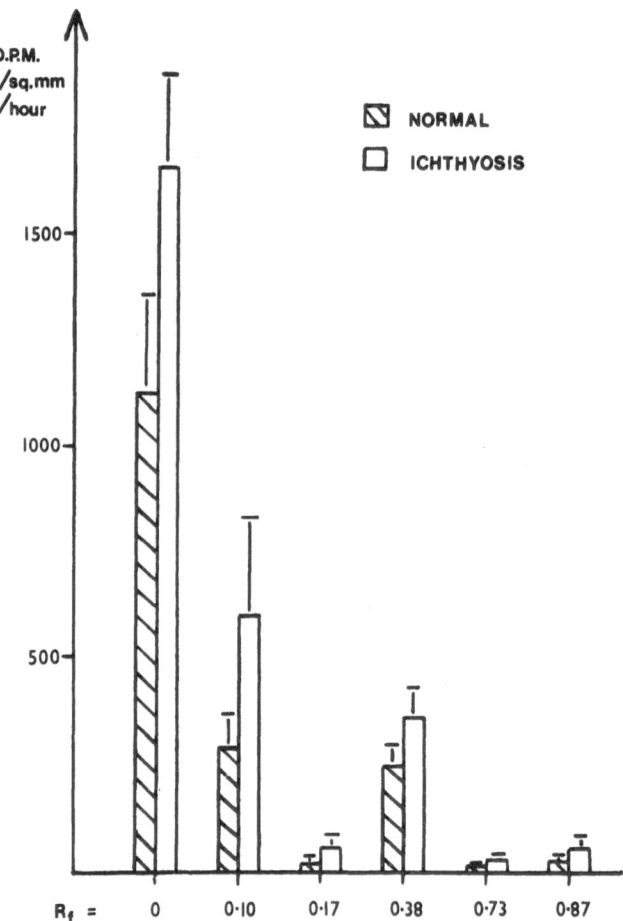

Figure 4.2 Pattern of incorporation of [¹⁴C]acetate in both normal (mean ± standard deviation, $n = 6$) and ichthyotic (mean ± standard deviation, $n = 7$) epidermis. Results are expressed as total d.p.m. per square mm per hour recovered in each of the six bands identified after development using the solvent system of Summerly and Woodbury[11]

Incorporation of ^{14}C acetate into individual lipid moieties

Lipid analysis

The radioactivities recoverable from each of the six bands detectable after development with the solvent system of Summerly and Woodbury are compared in Figure 4.2. Again an increased incorporation is apparent in the ichthyotic patients, compared to normal, in all bands recovered from the TLC plate. That the observed differences are also qualitative is demonstrated in Table 4.1. Here the results for each band are expressed as a percentage of

Table 4.1 TLC analysis of ^{14}C acetate containing lipids using the solvent system of Summerly and Woodbury

R_f	Provisional identity of radioactive band	Normals (n = 6)	Autosomal dominant ichthyosis (n = 7)	Refsum's disease (HAP)
0.00	Origin	66.2	61.0	55.8
0.10	Free sterol	16.7	21.5	39.8
0.17	Free fatty acids	0.8	2.0	0.6
0.38	Triglycerides	14.5	13.5	9.3
0.73	Sterol esters	0.4	0.5	0.6
0.87	Squalene	1.5	1.6	1.5

The results for each band are expressed as a percentage of the total radioactivity recoverable from the TLC plate.

the total recoverable radioactivity. An increase in the proportion of radioactivity in the free sterol band is observed in the ichthyotic group together with a decrease in the amount of material remaining at the origin. A similar but larger change is observed in the patient with Refsum's disease.

Phospholipid analysis

Apart from material running with the solvent front, five radioactive bands were

Table 4.2 TLC analysis of ^{14}C acetate containing phospholipids using the solvent system of Skipski, Peterson and Barclay

R_f	Provisional identity of radioactive bands	Normals (n = 6)	Autosomal dominant ichthyosis (n = 7)	Refsum's disease (HAP)
0.10	Lysophosphatidyl choline	2.3	2.2	4.7
0.21	Sphingomyelin	6.2	6.6	15.9
0.41	Phosphatidyl choline	35.6	39.0	42.5
0.58	Phosphatidyl serine	12.5	13.6	8.5
0.82	Phosphatidyl ethanolamine (?)	43.5	38.5	28.4

The results for each band are expressed as a percentage of the total radioactivity from the phospholipid bands.

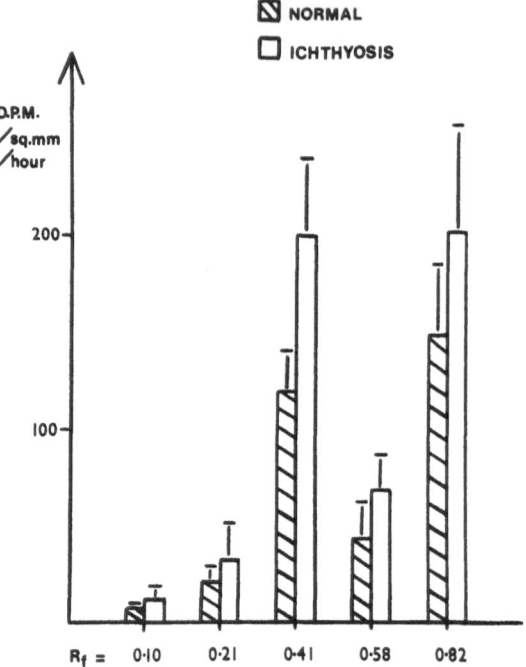

Figure 4.3 Pattern of [^{14}C]acetate in both normal (mean ± standard deviation, n = 6) and ichthyotic (mean ± standard deviation, $n = 7$) epidermis. Results are expressed as the total d.p.m. per square mm per hour recovered in each of the five radioactive phospholipid bands identified after development using the solvent system of Skipski, Peterson and Barclay[12]

detected using the solvent system of Skipski, Peterson and Barclay. The radioactivities recovered from each band for the ADI patients and normal individuals are given in Figure 4.3. Again an overall trend of increased incorporation of [^{14}C]acetate is observed in ichthyosis, although the only statistically significant difference was that associated with the phosphatidyl choline band ($P < 0.01$). When the results for each band are expressed as the percentage of the total phospholipid radioactivity (Table 4.2) it is again apparent that qualitative differences are observed. Thus phosphatidyl choline is increased in ADI compared to normal whereas phosphatidyl ethanolamine is decreased. Similar but larger differences relative to normal are again seen in Refsum's disease.

In vitro incorporation of [^{3}H]thymidine, proline and histidine

The *in vitro* rates of incorporation of tritiated precursors are given in Table 4.3. Whilst both thymidine and histidine did not differ significantly from normal, proline uptake was increased ($P < 0.01$).

Table 4.3 *In vitro* incorporation of radioactive precursors

	d.p.m. incorporated (per sq. mm. per hour)		
	Thymidine	*Proline*	*Histidine*
Normal range	96 ± 33 (n = 7)	240 ± 41 (n = 6)	107 ± 36 (n = 5)
Autosomal dominant ichthyosis patients (^{14}C Acetate study) (n = 7)	139 ± 50	524 ± 184	165 ± 72

DISCUSSION

Our preliminary findings indicate the following. Firstly that a quantitative difference exists in the rate of [^{14}C]acetate incorporation between ichthyotic and normal epidermis. Secondly that small qualitative differences also exist, in particular an increased incorporation into phosphatidyl choline.

The quantitative differences observed do not appear to be related to increased cell turnover. The *in vitro* uptake of tritiated thymidine is within normal range and the labelling index has been reported as normal[15,16] in this type of ichthyosis. However, abnormal protein synthesis may be occurring as evidenced by the high proline uptake and the importance of this in relation to lipogenesis is uncertain. The significance of increased uptake of ^{14}C acetate into the phosphatidyl choline fraction is a matter for speculation. Such incorporation is predominantly related to fatty acid synthesis and turnover which occurs independently of and more rapidly than phosphatidyl choline turnover as a whole. As such the difference observed may indicate an abnormality in plasma membrane biosynthesis which in itself may explain the abnormal desquamation. However, the fact that similar but larger changes occur in the epidermis in Refsum's disease suggests that these changes are not the primary abnormalities but are features of disordered desquamation. Investigation of non-ichthyotic disorders of desquamation may help resolve this question.

Acknowledgements

The authors are in receipt of a grant from the Wellcome Trust.

References

1. Achor, R. W. P., Winkelmann, R. K. and Perry, H. O. (1961). Cutaneous side effects from use of triparanol (Mer 29): Preliminary data on ichthyosis and loss of hair. *Proc. Mayo Clin.*, **36**, 217

2. Ruiter, M. and Meyler, L. (1960). Skin changes after therapeutic administration of nicotinic acid in large doses. *Dermatologica*, **120,** 139

3. Basnayake, V. and Sinclair, H. M. (1956). The effect of deficiency of essential fatty acids upon the skin. In: G. Popjak and E. LeBreton (eds.) *Biochemical Problems of Lipids.* p. 475. (London: Butterworth)

4. Press, M., Kikuchi, H., Shimoyama, T. and Thompson, G. R. (1974). Diagnosis and treatment of essential fatty acid deficiency in man. *Br. Med. J.*, **11,** 247

5. Kichterich, R., Van Mechelen, P. and Rossi, E. (1965). Refsum's disease (heredopathia atactica polyneuritiformis(: An inborn error of lipid metabolism with storage of 3,7,11,15-tetramethyl hexadecanoic acid. *Am. J. Med.*, **39,** 320

6. Malmendier, C. L., Jonniaux, G., Voet, W. and Van Den Bergen, C. J. (1974). Fatty acid composition of tissues in Refsum's disease (Heredopathia atactica polyneuritiformis). Estimation of total phytanic acid accumulation. *Biomedicine*, **20,** 398

7. Davies, M. G., Reynolds, D., Marks, R. and Dykes, P. J. (1977). The epidermis in Refsum's disease (Heredopathia Atactia Polyneuritiformis). *Presented at the 2nd Clinically Orientated Symposium of the European Society for Dermatological Research*, January 28, Welsh National School Of Medicine, Cardiff. (To be published)

8. Long, V. J. W. (1970). Variations in lipid composition at different depths in the cow snout epidermis. *J. Invest. Dermatol.*, **55,** 269

9. Gray, G. M. and Yardley, H. J. (1975). Different populations of pig epidermal cells: isolation and lipid composition. *J. Lipid Res.*, **16,** 441

10. Summerly, R. and Yardley, H. J. (1967). Cholesterol synthesis in ichthyosis vulgaris. *Br. J. Derm.*, **79,** 378

11. Summerly, R. and Woodbury, S. (1971). The *in vitro* incorporation of ¹⁴C-acetate into the isolated sebaceous gland and appendage free epidermis of human skin. *Br. J. Dermatol.*, **85,** 424

12. Skipski, V. P., Peterson, R. F. and Barclay, M. (1964). Quantitative analysis of phospholipids by thin layer chromatography. *Biochem. J.* **90,** 374

13. Marks, R., Fukui, K. and Halprin, K. (1971). The application of an *in vitro* technique to the study of epidermal replication and metabolism. *Br. J. Dermatol.*, **84,** 453

14. Holt, P. J. A. and Marks, R. (1976). Epidermal architecture, growth and metabolism in acromegaly. *Br. Med. J.*, **1,** 496

15. Frost, P. (1973). Ichthyosiform dermatoses. *J. Invest. Dermatol.*, **60,** 541

16. Marks, R. and Dykes, P. J. (1977). Epidermal growth characteristics in ichthyotic disorders. *Presented at the 2nd Clinically Orientated Symposium of the European Society for Dermatological Research*, January 28th, Welsh National School of Medicine, Cardiff. (To be published)

5
Immunofluorescence Studies in Ichthyosis Vulgaris

E. PANCONESI and P. FABBRI

INTRODUCTION

Among the most recent advances in the field of cutaneous immunopathology, those on psoriasis based on immunofluorescence research are of particular significance. These investigations have shown firstly, the presence of circulating complement-fixing autoantibodies directed specifically against the stratum corneum[1-5,7,8], secondly, that immunoglobulins (above all IgG, but also IgM and IgA) and the complement fraction C_3 are fixed to the stratum corneum[2,6,7,9,10,11]; and thirdly, that these fixed immunoglobulins can be identified with the circulating antibodies directed against the stratum corneum[9,10].

During our current research on the immunopathology of psoriasis we have also paid special attention to various keratinization disorders, in particular ichthyosis vulgaris. This has provided us with interesting material for comparative studies.

MATERIALS AND METHODS

Skin biopsies were performed on 15 subjects with ichthyosis vulgaris. The specimens were taken from the extensor surface of the forearm and examined both by direct immunofluorescence (D.If.) and by the *four compartment system*. The D.If. technique has been described in our previous studies[12,13]. The characteristics of the antisera used are referred to in detail in Table 5.1.

The *four compartment system* is a particular combination of immuno-fluorescence tests adopted by Jablonska et al.[10] for the proper immunological study of the stratum corneum. Each biopsy specimen was subjected to a

Table 5.1 Characteristics of conjugates

Antisera	anti-IgG	anti-IgA	anti-IgM	anti-C$_3$	anti-Fibrinogen
Molar F/P	3.0	2.3	3.3	2.3	2.1
Molar Ab/P	0.079	0.093	0.093	0.16	—
Molar Ab/F	0.026	0.041	0.028	0.07	—

special series of tests so that the specificity and reproducibility of the results were ensured (see Table 5.2). In the first two compartments the anti-IgG conjugate (dilution 1:128) is adsorbed with a normal serum to remove anti-IgG antibodies so that any eventual non-specific reactions to the fluorochrome

Table 5.2 Example of use of the 'four-compartment system' for one biopsy

Compartment	Section number	Immunofluorescence test (each section was examined by UV and BV light)	
1st	1 5	PBS	Anti-IgG conjugate adsorbed with normal human serum
2nd	3 7	1/10 dilution of serum with a SC Ab titre <80 (serum No. 1567)	(diluted 1/128)
3rd	2 6 9	PBS	Anti-IgG conjugate diluted 1/32 to contain 1/8 U anti-IgG antibody
4th	4 8 10	1/10 dilution of serum with a SC Ab titre <80 (serum No. 1567)	

would be noted. The third compartment reports the D.If. findings, and these are then compared in the fourth compartment with the fluorescence findings obtained by applying to the same section (which acts as an antigenic substrate) the serum from a psoriatic containing a high titre — 1:80 — of anti-stratum corneum antibodies. The anti-IgG conjugate was diluted 1:32 to contain 1/8 U (equalling 25 μg/ml) of anti-IgG antibody (see Table 5.2).

A third series of experiments was done to check the eventual modifications of the intercellular substance (i.s.) in the Malpighian layer and stratum corneum. The antigenic substrate of five of the ichthyotic subjects was treated with serum with anti-i.s. antibodies (titre 1:320) taken from a pemphigus patient (see Figure 5.1). Each section was treated with two different dilutions of pemphigus serum (1:10 and 1:40) and with an anti-IgG conjugate (same characteristics as above).

The specimens were examined with a Leitz Orthoplan fluorescence incident light microscope fitted with an Osram HBO 200 W mercury bulb. The exciter filters used were BG 38 and K 480 + 2KP 490; the dichroic mirror was TK

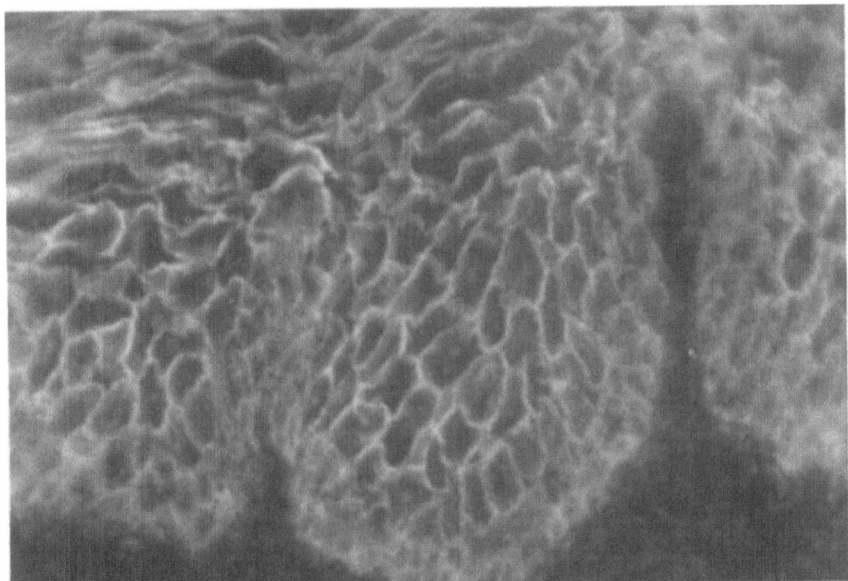

Figure 5.1 Fluorescence micrograph to show positive I.S. staining in ichthyotic epidermis with pemphigus serum

510, and the barrier filters were K 515 + K 510. In the *four compartment* experiments each specimen was examined with two light systems, ultraviolet and blue-violet. The filters used with the blue-violet light were BG 12 and KP 490 × 2.

Immunofluorescence was recorded photographically on Kodak Ektachrome high-speed film.

RESULTS

Our findings can be summarized as follows (see Table 5.3).

1. The immunoglobulins and complement do not fix to the stratum corneum of subjects with ichthyosis vulgaris.

2. Anti-stratum corneum antibodies fix to their specific antigens (see Figure 5.2) in varying ways. Sometimes they give intercellular fluorescence, sometimes cytoplasmic.

Table 5.3 Results obtained with the 'four-compartment system' in 15 cases of ichthyosis vulgaris

1st Compartment	No IF staining
2nd Compartment	No IF staining
3rd Compartment	No IF staining
4th Compartment	IF staining

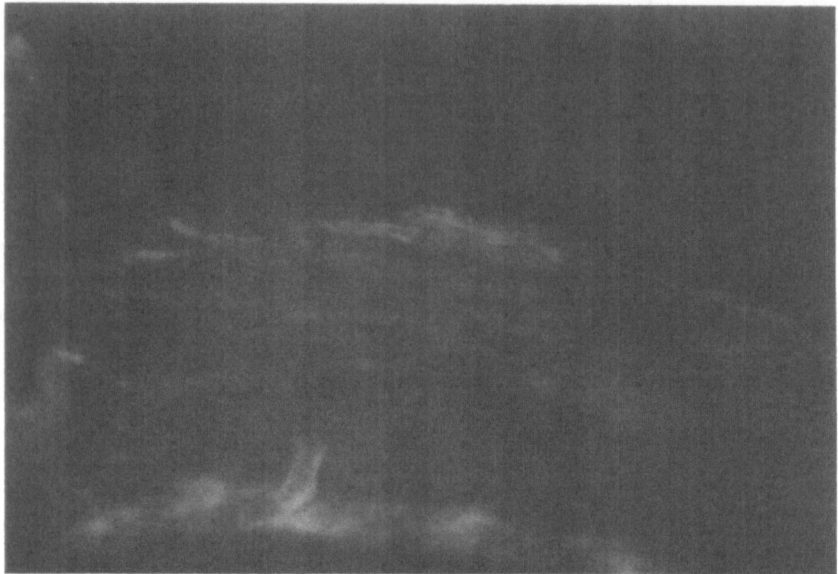

Figure 5.2   Fluorescence micrograph to show positive staining in ichthyotic stratum corneum

3. Pemphigus antibodies fix to the i.s. in both the Malpighian layer and the stratum corneum (see Table 5.4). It should be noted that the intensity of the fluorescence varies considerably from one substrate to another; it also diminishes in relation to the dilution of the serum.

Table 5.4   Results obtained with pemphigus antibodies on skin biopsies in five cases of ichthyosis vulgaris

Case No.	Titre of pemphigus serum used	Immunofluorescence result	
		IS staining of str. corneum	IS staining of str. Malpighii
1	1/10	++	++
	1/40	+	+
2	1/10	+	++
	1/40	(+)	(+)
3	1/10	++	++
	1/40	+	+
4	1/10	+	+
	1/40	+	+
5	1/10	++	++
	1/40	++	++

DISCUSSION

This immunopathological study using D.If. and other immunological methods not reported here (the dosage of the Ig of the various complement fractions, the search for non-organ specific antibodies) documents the lack of involvement of immunologic mechanisms, even secondary ones, in the pathogenesis of ichthyosis vulgaris. Furthermore, the disease itself does not apparently provoke any modifications in the antigenic characteristics of the stratum corneum, which appear essentially identical to those of normal epidermis. Our investigations also permit us to point out that the antigenic characteristics of the i.s. are not altered in either the stratum Malpighii or stratum corneum.

References

1. Krogh, H. K. and Tonder, O. (1968). Adherence of erythrocytes to stratum corneum of skin tissue sections. *Int. Arch. Allergy App. Immunol.*, **34**, 170
2. Krogh, H. K. (1968). Role of complement in the adherence of erythrocytes to stratum corneum. *Int. Arch. Allergy App. Immunol.*, **34**, 397
3. Krogh, H. K. (1969). Antibodies in human sera to stratum corneum. *Int. Arch. Allergy. App. Immunol.*, **36**, 415
4. Krogh, H. K. (1970). Low molecular weight antibodies in human sera to stratum corneum. *Int. Arch. Allergy. App. Immunol.*, **37**, 104
5. Krogh, H. K. (1970). The occurrence of antibodies to stratum corneum in man. *Int. Arch. Allergy App. Immunol.*, **37**, 649
6. Krogh, H. K. and Tonder, O. (1972). Immunoglobulins and anti-immunoglobulin factors in psoriatic lesions. *Clin. Exp. Immunol.*, **10**, 623
7. Krogh, H. K. and Tonder, O. (1973). Antibodies in psoriatic scales. *Scand. J. Immunol.*, **2**, 45
8. Beutner, E. H., Jablonska, S., Jarrabek-Chorzelska, M., Maciejowska, E., Rzesa, G. and Chorzelski, T. P. (1975). Studies in immunodermatology. VI. I.F. studies of autoantibody to the stratum corneum of psoriatic lesions. *Int. Arch. Allergy App. Immunol.*, **48**, 301
9. Beutner, E. H., Chorzelski, T. P. and Jablonska, S. (1976). Studies on possible significance of the universal stratum corneum antibodies in the pathogenesis of psoriasis. Paper read at the 2nd International Symposium at Stanford. (In press.)
10. Jablonska, S., Chorzelski, T. P., Jarrabek Chorzelska, M. and Beutner, E. H. (1976). Studies in immunodermatology. VII. Four-compartment system studies of IgG in stratum corneum antigen in biopsies of psoriasis and control dermatoses. *Int. Arch. Allergy App. Immunol.*, **48**, 324
11. Guilhou, J. J., Clot, J., Meynadier, J. and Lapinski, H. (1976). Immunological aspects of psoriasis. I. Immunoglobulins and anti-IgG factors. *Br. J. Derm.*, **94**, 501
12. Panconesi, E. (1974). La Patogenesi autoimmune in dermatologia (Cap. 4, Fabbri, P. 'Ricerche di immunopatologia cutanea nel pemfigo, nei pemfigoidi, nel lupus erythematosus'). *53° Congresso SIDES*, Rome, October 1974
13. Fabbri, P., DePalma, A. and Giannotti, B. (1975). Unusual findings with direct immunofluorescence examination in dermatitis herpetiformis. *Ital. Gen. Rev. Derm.*, **2** (serie 2°), 9

6
Growth Characteristics of the Epidermis in the Ichthyotic Disorders

R. MARKS and P. J. DYKES

INTRODUCTION

In comparison with psoriasis the ichthyoses have commanded relatively little attention from researchers as far as the population dynamics of the epidermis are concerned. Frost[1] and Fisher and Wells[2] found no serious disturbance of the rate of epidermal cell production in autosomal dominant ichthyosis. However, a high rate of epidermopoiesis was noted in non-bullous ichthyosiform erythroderma by Frost[1].

Our own studies have concerned the following groups of patients with 'ichthyotic' conditions.

(a) Autosomal dominant ichthyosis
(b) patients with non-bullous ichthyosiform erythroderma
(c) patients with a marked hyperkeratosis as part of their disorder and who have been variously designated in the past but who we describe as 'lamellar ichthyosis'
(d) patients with acquired ichthyosis and
(e) one patient with Refsum's syndrome.

PATIENTS AND METHODS

Patients with autosomal dominant ichthyosis (ADI) fulfilled the usual clinical criteria for this disorder[1] — (five men, four women, mean age = 40.5 years). The two patients with non-bullous ichthyosiform erythroderma are briefly

Table 6.1 Clinical details of patients studied with non-bullous ichthyosiform erythroderma and lamellar ichthyosis

Patient	Age	Sex	Diagnosis	Main clinical characteristics
1*	72	M	lamellar ichthyosis	Large shield like polygonal scales on limbs. Marked hyperkeratosis at times. Sparse hair, 'crumpled ears', ectropion
2	34	M	lamellar ichthyosis	Similar clinical picture to patient '1' but less severe
3*	54	F	ichthyosiform erythroderma	Fine prolific scaling and generalized erythema. Ectropion
4	26	M	ichthyosiform erythroderma	Generally similar to patient '3' but linear hyperkeratotic areas in antecubital and popliteal fossae and marked plantar hyperkeratosis

* Patients 1 and 3 have been presented elsewhere[6].

described in Table 6.1 as are the two patients with 'lamellar ichthyosis'. The patients with acquired ichthyosis are described in Table 6.2, and the patient with Refsum's syndrome has already been described in this symposium (Chapter 8). The methods that we have used to estimate the rates of epidermal cell production have been of two types. Firstly we have employed an *in vitro* technique to determine the rates of thymidine incorporation based on that of Marks *et al.* (1971)[3] and described in more detail by Holt and Marks (1976)[4]. Essentially this technique depends on the incubation of skin fragments in the presence of tritiated thymidine. These fragments were obtained from the lateral aspect of the thigh using a Castroviejo keratotome set at 0.4 mm. At the end of incubation the fragments (consisting predominantly of epidermis) were washed, homogenized and the macromolecules precipitated with perchloric acid. The solubilized precipitate was counted in a scintillation counter and the activities of each fragment expressed as d.p.m./sq. mm of explant area/h incubation. Each result represents the mean of three observations.

The second technique employed also utilizes the uptake of tritiated thymidine by the epidermal nuclei during the synthetic phase of the mitotic cycle and is basically an autoradiographic method. The tritiated thymidine was either injected intracutaneously *in vivo* (10 μCi in 0.1 ml saline, Sp. Act. 18–21 Ci/mmol, Amersham) or presented to the tissue *in vitro*. In the latter situation the incubation was either for four hours (keratotome fragments, 1 μCi/ml specific activity 2 Ci/mmol) or 2.5 hours under the conditions described by Shahrad and Marks[5]. The autoradiographs were prepared according to standard methods using Ilford nuclear emulsion (K2). Labelling indices were derived from the autoradiographs by counting the labelled basal and suprabasal cells and expressing them as a percentage of a total of 1000 basal cells.

Table 6.2 Clinical details of patients with acquired ichthyosis

Patient	Age	Sex	Underlying systemic disorder	Skin condition
5*	60	M	Alcoholism, malnutrition	Widespread dryness and scaliness most marked on limbs
6*	57	M	Reticulum cell sarcoma	Widespread dryness and scaliness. Slight pinkness in background
7*	15	M	None found	Severe dryness and shield-like scaling. Most marked on limbs and back
8*	61	M	Pan hypopituitarism	Dry, scaly skin, loss of body hair. Intermittently severe. Large white polygonal scales
9†	62	M	Crohns disease	Generalized dryness and slight scaliness
10†	53	M	Post partial gastrectomy for peptic ulcer	Generalized dryness and slight scaliness
11†	53	M	Crohns disease	Generalized dryness and slight scaliness
12†	5	M	Coeliac disease	Generalized dryness and slight scaliness
13†	54	F	Crohns disease	Generalized dryness and slight scaliness
14†	68	M	Proctocolitis	Generalized dryness and slight scaliness
15†	67	M	Post partial gastrectomy	Generalized dryness and slight scaliness
16†	42	M	Coeliac disease	Generalized dryness and slight scaliness
17†	44	F	Ileo jejunal by-pass for obesity	Generalized dryness and slight scaliness

* Patients 5–8 have been presented elsewhere[7].
† Patients 9–17 have been presented elsewhere[8].

In some cases the epidermal architecture was recorded quantitatively by determining,

(a) the epidermal thickness (in numbers of viable cells) at 20 random sites, and
(b) the ratio of the length of the basal layer to that of the granular cell layer. (B/G ratio).

RESULTS

The rates of thymidine incorporation for the various types of ichthyotic

Table 6.3 Results of thymidine incorporation in patients with various types of ichthyosis

Type of ichthyosis	Number of patients (or patient number from Table 2)	Thymidine incorporation
Normal values	10	99 ± 32*
Autosomal dominant ichthyosis	9	131 ± 46*
Patients with malabsorption	9	96 ± 51*
Acquired ichthyosis	Patient Number 8	103*
Refsum's disease	1	444*
Normal values	24	12 ± 7.7†
Lamellar ichthyosis	2	3.2† (1.8, 4.3)
Ichthyosiform erythroderma	2	34.9† (24.6, 45.2)

Results are expressed as d.p.m. incorporated per square mm skin surface per hour incubation ± standard deviation* or as corrected counts per minute as defined by Marks, Fukui and Halprin (1971)†.

conditions are given in Table 6.3. The results of labelling index studies are given in Table 6.4 and epidermal measurements are given in Table 6.5.

COMMENT

Clearly the patients with ichthyosiform erythroderma and Refsum's disease are different with regard to the rate of cell proliferation from the bulk of patients with ichthyotic disorders. It is perhaps not quite so surprising that those with ichthyosiform erythroderma have a high rate of epidermal cell division as their skin is reddened and 'inflamed' and could be difficult to distinguish clinically from patients with universal psoriasis. It is, however, surprising that the patient with Refsum's syndrome had such a high rate of epidermal cell production in our autoradiographic and thymidine incorporation experiments. It is of considerable interest in this respect that essential fatty acid (EFA) deficient

Table 6.4 Labelling index measurement for the ichthyotic disorders

Type of ichthyosis	In vitro/in vivo measurement	No. of patients (or patient number from Table 2)	Labelling index ± standard deviation
Autosomal dominant ichthyosis	In vitro	9	3.9 ± 1.3*
Refsum's syndrome	In vitro/in vivo	1	16.3*, 22.0†
Acquired ichthyosis	In vitro	Number 5	3.0*
Acquired ichthyosis	In vitro	Number 7	8.4‡
Acquired ichthyosis	In vitro	Number 8	5.8*
Patients with malabsorption	In vitro	4	3.2 ± 1.1*

* Normal range 3.8 ± 1.0 (n = 5).
† Normal range 5.1 ± 0.8 (n = 25).
‡ Normal range 8.4 ± 2.1 (n = 9).

Table 6.5   Results of epidermal measurements in the ichthyotic disorders

Type of ichthyotic disorder	Number of patients (or patient number)	Mean B/G ratio ± standard deviation	Mean epidermal thickness ± standard deviation
Autosomal dominant ichthyosis	6	1.2 ± 0.2	5.2 ± 1.0
Lamellar ichthyosis	Patients 1, 2	1.3, 1.5	6.0, 9.7
Ichthyosiform erythroderma	Patients 2, 4	2.3, 2.2	19.4, 12.0
Acquired ichthyosis	Patients 5, 7, 8	1.1, 1.5, 1.0	4.8, 6.9, 3.8
Refsum's syndrome	1	1.2	6.8
Normal range		1.2 ± 0.1	5.1 ± 1.2

animals also have a similarly high labelling index (see Chapter 2) and that their epidermis is also characterized by hyperkeratosis and hypergranulosis.

It may be that the defect in the plasma membrane phospholipids presumably produced by the EFA deficiency is similar to an abnormality produced by the displacement of linoleic and arachidonic acids by the excess phytanic acid in Refsum's syndrome and that there is a special relationship between the plasma membrane and cell division. The normal rate of cell production in dominant ichthyosis that we have found is in agreement with previous workers and the scaliness in these patients is an optical and sensory effect from the abnormal type of desquamation in these patients rather than an increase in scale production. We believe that the hyperkeratotic type of lamellar ichthyosis is 'special' in that there is a normal or low rate of cell production in contra-distinction to the erythrodermatous types.

It seems that it is not cell production that is at fault in any of the ichthyotic disorders that we have studied, but that any deviation in this function is consequent on the disturbed metabolism of the keratinizing portion of the epidermis.

References

1. Frost, P. (1973). Ichthyosiform dermatoses. *J. Invest. Dermatol.*, **60**, 541
2. Fisher, L. B. and Wells, G. C. (1968). The mitotic rate and duration of lesions in psoriasis and ichthyosis. *Br. J. Dermatol.*, **84**, 235
3. Marks, R., Fukui, K. and Halprin, K. (1971). The application of an *in vitro* technique to the study of epidermal replication and metabolism. *Br. J. Dermatol.*. **84**, 453
4. Holt, P. J. A. and Marks, R. (1976). Epidermal architecture, growth and metabolism in acromegaly. *Br. Med. J.*, **1**, 496
5. Shahrad, P. and Marks, R. (1976). Hair follicle kinetics in psoriasis. *Br. J. Dermatol.*, **94**, 7
6. Delaney, T. J., Marks, R. and Gold, S. C. (1973). Congenital ichthyosiform erythroderma and lamellar ichthyosis: two patients contrasted. *Proc. R. Soc. Med.*, **66**, 1173

7. Dykes, P. J. and Marks, R. (1977). Acquired ichthyosis. Multiple causes for an acquired generalised disturbance in desquamation. *Br. J. Dermatol.* **97,** 327

8. Dykes, P. J. and Marks, R. (1977). Epidermal lipogenesis and macromolecular synthesis in autosomal dominant ichthyosis and the 'acquired ichthyosis' associated with disorders of the small bowel. (Presented at the annual meeting of the European Society for Dermatological Research, May 2–4, Amsterdam)

7
The Proteins of Epidermis in Relation to Normal and Abnormal Keratinization

D. SKERROW

BOVINE EPIDERMIS

This work involves the application to normal and abnormal human epidermis of some biochemical techniques which were originally developed for bovine epidermis. The biochemical study of epidermal keratinization was revolutionized by the discovery that citric acid–sodium citrate (CASC) buffer, pH 2.6, is capable of dispersing the living cells of cow's nose epidermis and, from the CASC extract, the fibrous protein prekeratin can be isolated[1,2].

Prekeratin is the protein of the epidermal tonofilaments and the bovine material has now been characterized in some detail[3,4]. Many features of its molecular architecture are known and, most importantly for the purposes of this study, it has been shown to consist of three different polypeptide chains which can be readily detected on sodium dodecyl sulphate (SDS)-polyacrylamide gels.

The ability to recognize the three chains of the fibrous protein, and to be certain of their origin, made it possible, for the first time, to begin answering some very simple but fundamental questions about keratinization. For example: does this molecule become chemically modified during keratinization? Does it become cross-linked by disulphide bonds or do the molecular weights of its chains become altered? The answer to each of these questions appears to be no. It is possible to take cow's nose stratum corneum and extract it with neutral 6M urea with no reducing agent to break disulphide bonds. When this is done and the extract run on SDS-polyacrylamide gels, about 60% of the weight of the stratum corneum is recovered in the form of fibrous protein chains which are of identical mobilities to those of prekeratin

43

LIVING CELLS
cow's nose epidermis

| CASC buffer,
| pH 2.6

PREKERATIN
3-chain protein

CORNIFIED CELLS
cow's nose epidermis

| urea buffer,
| pH 7, no reducing agent

'PREKERATIN' CHAINS
accounting for 60% of
weight of stratum corneum

Figure 7.1   Extraction of living and cornified cow's nose epidermal cells. The three chains of prekeratin, extracted by CASC pH 2.6, from the tonofilaments of living cells can be identified by SDS-gel electrophoresis. The use of 6M urea, combined with efficient homogenization of the cornified cells by a French pressure cell[5] or Polytron homogenizer[6] releases about 60% of the weight of the stratum corneum in the form of 'prekeratin' chains indistinguishable from those in the living cells. As the homogenization and subsequent gel runs are performed without the use of a reducing agent it is apparent that the prekeratin chains are not modified during keratinization by the introduction of inter-chain disulphide or other covalent cross-links. Similar results to this have now been obtained for human epidermis, although the yield of 'prekeratin' chains from the stratum corneum has not yet been fully quantified

from the living cells[5,6] (Figure 7.1). So the fibrous protein of bovine epidermis is not detectably modified during keratinization by the introduction of disulphide or other covalent cross-links.

NORMAL HUMAN EPIDERMIS

With this background from bovine epidermis it was possible to determine whether these techniques can be applied to human epidermis and whether any

Table 7.1   Amino acid compositions* of human and bovine prekeratin

Amino acid	Human prekeratin	Bovine prekeratin[8]
Cysteic acid	13.3	8.8
Aspartic acid	87.2	89.5
Threonine	43.9	35.3
Serine	108.9	93.6
Glutamic acid	119.2	143.5
Proline	22.7	14.9
Glycine	173.8	157.0
Alanine	53.5	67.6
Valine	49.8	51.4
Methionine	8.8	20.4
Isoleucine	45.9	41.0
Leucine	86.8	87.9
Tyrosine	26.7	27.7
Phenylalanine	36.3	37.5
Lysine	54.6	52.1
Histidine	14.4	8.8
Arginine	53.9	58.6

* Expressed as residues/1000. Corrected for the destruction and slow release of residues.

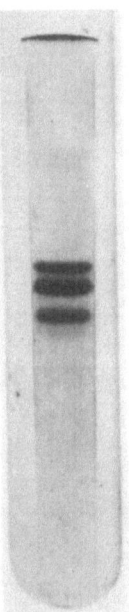

Figure 7.2 SDS-polyacrylamide gel electrophoresis of human prekeratin. Human prekeratin was prepared by modifying the CASC, pH 2.6, procedure used for bovine prekeratin and then subjected to SDS-gel electrophoresis on 7.5% acrylamide gels[7]. The three polypeptide chains of human prekeratin are resolved and have estimated molecular weights of 70 000, 63 000 and 55 000. The chain molecular weights are unaltered if the prekeratin is reduced prior to application to the gels, demonstrating the absence of interchain disulphide bonds in this molecule

detectable abnormalities are present in pathological conditions in which keratinization may be affected. It was found possible to apply the CASC extraction and isolation procedures, with suitable modifications, to human epidermis and to isolate human prekeratin. This is very similar to the bovine material. It has three chains of about the same molecular weights as the bovine, which are shown separated in Figure 7.2. These again have no disulphide bonds between them and their overall amino acid composition is very similar to that of bovine prekeratin (Table 7.1), suggesting that much of the more sophisticated work with the bovine molecule will apply to the human.

This protein, as extracted with CASC, is derived from the living cells but, having purified it and determined that these chains are derived from it, it is again possible to look at total extracts of horny cells obtained by other reagents such as neutral 6M urea. When this is done with normal human callus, the same three chains are again obtained as are obtained from the living cells. So, there is no detectable difference between the fibrous protein of the tono-filaments seen in the cytoplasm of living cells (Figure 7.3A) and the filaments in horny cells which have become embedded in an electron-dense matrix and surrounded by a thickened and convoluted cell envelope (Figures 7.3B and

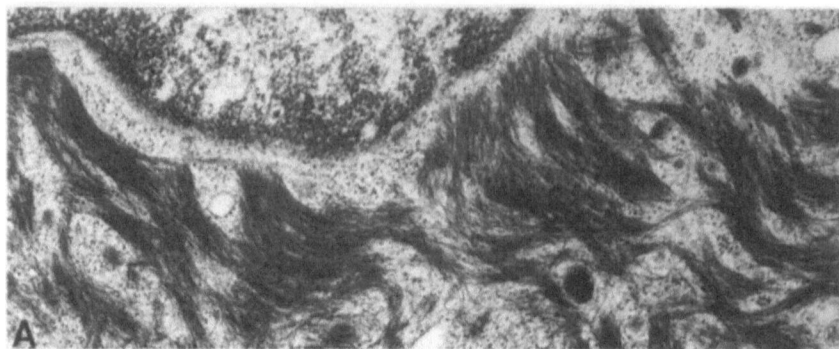

Figure 7.3A Portion of basal cell, with nucleus at upper left, showing numerous filament bundles in longitudinal section (×22 000)

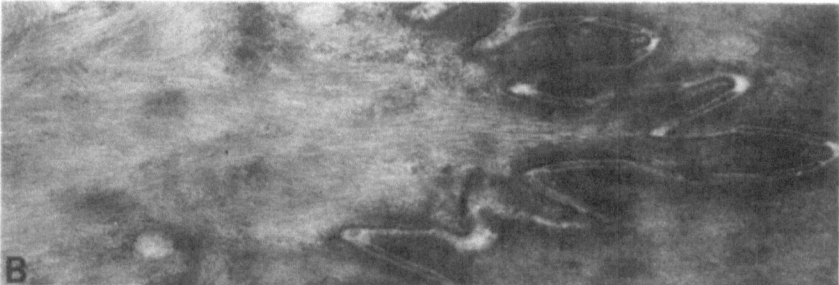

Figure 7.3B Two interdigitating normal horny cells occupied solely by filaments and matrix and surrounded by highly convoluted thickened cell envelopes. Most of the filaments are seen in longitudinal section (×36 080)

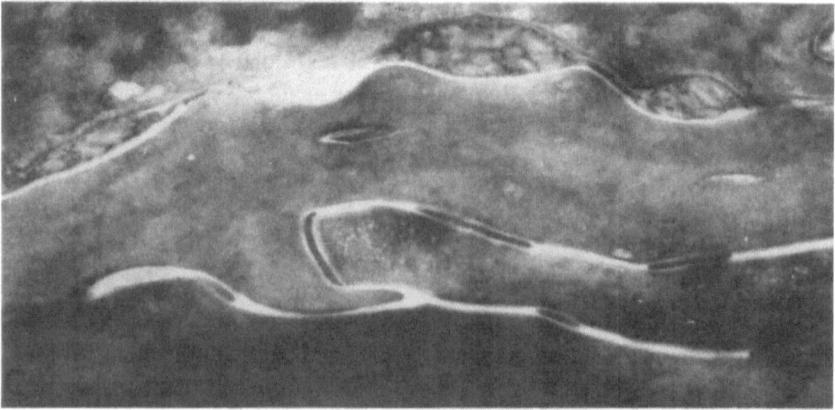

Figure 7.3C Portions of several normal horny cells, showing the 'speckled' appearance produced by the filaments in transverse section (×33 440)

7.3C). Whatever covalent cross-linking occurs during keratinization must, then, be around and about the filaments rather than involving them directly.

ABNORMAL HUMAN EPIDERMIS

Electron microscopy

Electron microscopy of the stratum corneum does not give the ability to distinguish between the proteins produced during normal keratinization and those of psoriatic and ichthyotic scale. In psoriatic scale (Figure 7.4A),

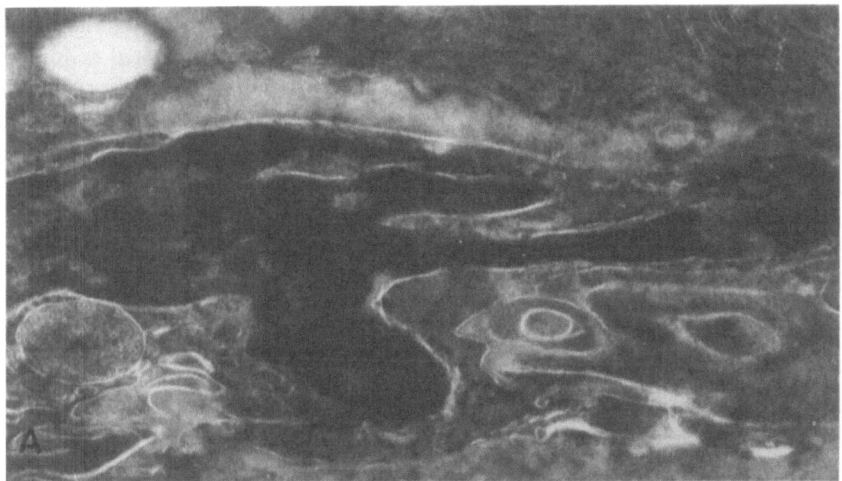

Figure 7.4A Portions of parakeratotic cells in psoriatic scale containing remnants of nuclei and other organelles. Between these inclusions, the filaments, seen here in transverse section, and matrix are apparently normal ($\times$40 480)

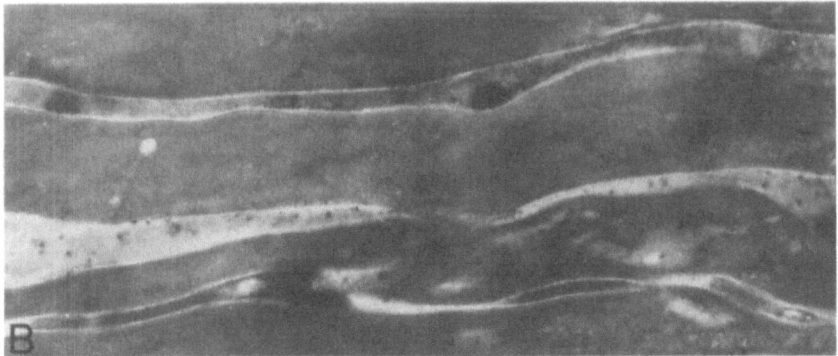

Figure 7.4B Cells from ichthyotic scale. No retained organelles are present and the cell contents closely resemble those of normal horny layer ($\times$40 480)

47

although the parakeratotic nuclei and lipid droplets typical of this condition are readily seen, high magnification of the cell contents only shows a filament-matrix complex which is not readily distinguishable from normal. In ichthyotic scale (Figure 7.4B) from autosomal dominant ichthyosis vulgaris the appearance is completely normal with the filament-matrix complex not being interrupted by the retained organelles and lipid droplets as in psoriasis.

Extraction and SDS-gel electrophoresis

However, being able to extract the constituent polypeptide chains of the stratum corneum proteins and separate them on gels allows us, for the first time, to compare in detail the terminal protein composition of normal and pathological epidermis at the molecular level. The first pathological condition to be examined in this way was psoriasis. When extracts of psoriatic scale are compared with those from normal epidermis or callus, a quite distinct difference is visible (Figure 7.5). Whereas the normal shows all of the three chains of the fibrous protein, in the psoriatic scale the uppermost or heaviest molecular weight chain is either virtually or completely absent. This chain is, however, present in the uninvolved callus of psoriatics and, during treatment, can be seen to increase in scales taken consecutively from the same lesion.

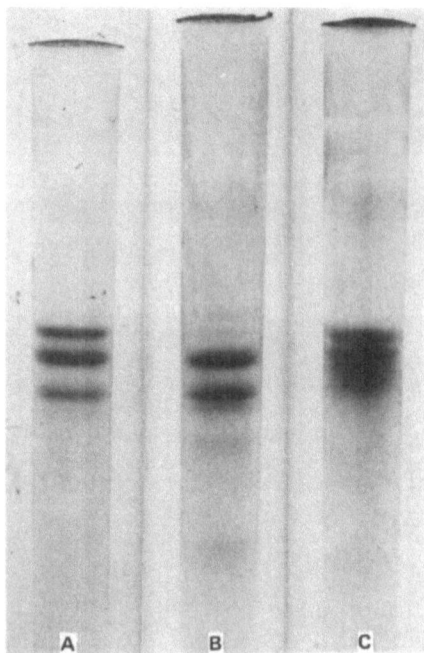

Figure 7.5 Comparison of extracts of A, normal callus B, psoriatic scale and C, ichthyotic scale. Each extract was obtained by homogenizing in neutral 6M urea/1% 2-mercaptoethanol then treated with SDS and run on 7.5% acrylamide gels containing SDS[7]

There are three possible general reasons for the absence of this chain from psoriatic scale. The first is that it is not synthesized. The second is that it is synthesized but then digested away by proteolytic enzyme activity during the abnormal keratinization process. The third is that it is synthesized but then becomes covalently cross-linked during the abnormal keratinization and is thus not extracted by the reagents used.

Although it is impossible to rule out any of these possibilities, it seems unlikely that the psoriatic cell, which is involved in an accelerated keratinization process with less than normal digestion of the cell organelles would either elaborate an additional cross-link or digest away one of these chains in a specific manner. So the most likely explanation at present is that one chain is not synthesized and there is, in fact, a gross molecular defect in the psoriatic fibrous protein.

In the case of ichthyotic scale, obtained from autosomal dominant ichthyosis vulgaris, however, a much more normal gel pattern is obtained (Figure 7.5). The uppermost band, which is absent in psoriatic scale, is clearly present. The lower two bands appear to travel as three. This is probably not significant as this appearance is occasionally given by normal callus extracts and seems to result from technical difficulties in processing dilute solutions.

Amino acid analysis

The same general picture of the protein composition of psoriatic and ichthyotic scale emerges from examination of their amino acid compositions (Table 7.2).

Table 7.2 Amino acid compositions* of psoriatic scale, normal callus and ichthyotic scale

Amino acid	Psoriatic scale	Callus	Ichthyotic scale
Cysteic acid	27.0	13.6	23.2
Aspartic acid	87.8	76.8	72.6
Threonine	54.3	38.6	37.6
Serine	81.5	145.8	145.9
Glutamic acid	118.5	121.7	123.0
Proline	56.7	22.3	36.9
Glycine	90.9	208.7	222.7
Alanine	65.3	39.2	42.1
Valine	60.7	34.9	38.0
Methionine	16.0	10.2	4.9
Isoleucine	47.1	36.4	33.8
Leucine	85.2	61.0	67.2
Tyrosine	35.8	33.9	30.0
Phenylalanine	35.6	28.0	30.8
Lysine	70.6	61.0	47.5
Histidine	20.3	20.2	15.2
Arginine	46.4	47.7	29.6

* Expressed as residues/1000. Corrected for the destruction and slow release of residues.

Taking into account the fact that these analyses are of whole tissues rather than purified proteins, it is possible to see that psoriatic scale has a generally similar overall amino acid composition to that of normal callus except for two residues—glycine and serine. These are very much reduced in the psoriatic scale with most of the other residues being relatively increased in order to compensate for this. However, the ichthyotic scale again appears to be more nearly normal as regards its protein composition. The glycine and serine levels are normal and none of the other amino acids differ significantly from normal.

CONCLUSIONS

The use of SDS-polyacrylamide gel electrophoresis, combined with the ability to recognize on the gels the fibrous protein chains of the tonofilaments provides a powerful tool for studying keratinization. It has been shown by this technique that, during normal keratinization, the fibrous protein does not become cross-linked by interchain disulphide bonds or other covalent cross-links. In psoriatic scale, it has been shown that the fibrous protein appears grossly abnormal, being deficient in one polypeptide chain. This is paralleled in psoriatic scale by a large decrease in the amounts of glycine and serine present. In ichthyotic scale, no such defect has, so far, been identified and it appears that any gross abnormality in ichthyosis must reside elsewhere than in the protein of the tonofilaments.

Acknowledgements

I wish to thank Dr. Christine J. Skerrow for producing the electron micrographs in this study. The work was supported by a grant from the Medical Research Council.

References

1. Matoltsy, A. G. (1964). Prekeratin. *Nature (London)*, **201,** 1130
2. Matoltsy, A. G. (1965). Soluble prekeratin. In A. G. Lyne and B. F. Short (eds.). *Biology of the Skin and Hair Growth*, p. 291 (Sydney: Angus and Robertson)
3. Skerrow, D., Matoltsy, A. G. and Matoltsy, M. N. (1973). Isolation and characterization of the α-helical regions of epidermal prekeratin. *J. Biol. Chem.*, **248,** 4820
4. Skerrow, D. (1974). The structure of prekeratin. *Biochem. Biophys. Res. Commun.*, **59,** 1311
5. Skerrow, D. (1973). Unpublished results
6. Steinert, P. M. (1975). The extraction and characterization of bovine epidermal α-keratin. *Biochem. J.*, **149,** 39
7. Weber, K. and Osborn, M. (1969). The reliability of molecular weight determinations by dodecyl sulfate–polyacrylamide gel electrophoresis. *J. Biol. Chem.*, **244,** 4406
8. Skerrow, D. (1972). A repeating subunit of soluble prekeratin. *Biochem. Biophys. Acta.*, **257,** 398

8
The Epidermis in Refsum's Disease (Heredopathia Atactica Polyneuritiformis)

M. G. DAVIES, D. J. REYNOLDS, R. MARKS and P. J. DYKES

INTRODUCTION

Heredopathia atactica polyneuritiformis (HAP, Refsum's Disease) comprises retinitis pigmentosa, peripheral polyneuropathy, cerebellar ataxia, deafness and ichthyosis as its major clinical components. It is extremely rare and shows an autosomal recessive mode of inheritance. It was first described by Refsum in 1946[1]. There were no real advances in our understanding of the disease until 1963 when Klenk and Kahlke[2] found high concentrations of an unusual branched chain C_{20} fatty acid (3,7,11,15-tetramethylhexadecanoic acid or phytanic acid) in renal and hepatic lipids and in the urine of an affected patient. This suggested a biochemical defect and subsequently phytanic acid in relatively large amounts was found in the blood of patients with Refsum's disease[3]. (It occurs normally in human plasma in very low concentrations — 0.4–2 μg/ml representing less than 0.1% of total fatty acids[4].)

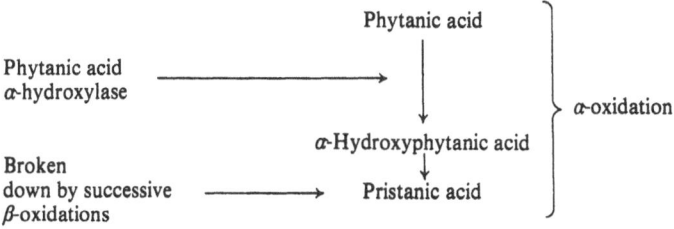

Figure 8.1 Biochemical pathway for the conversion of phytanic acid to pristanic acid

It has been shown that patients with Refsum's disease do not synthesize phytanic acid[5-7]. This strongly suggested an exogenous origin for the phytanic acid and both phytol and phytanic acid itself were shown to be potential dietary sources when fed in large doses to experimental animals[8]. The normal pathway for the degradation of phytanic acid was established by Steinberg and co-workers[9] and is shown in Figure 8.1. Conversion to pristanic acid by α-oxidation is an essential step before sequential β-oxidation can take place.

Cell culture studies[10-12] indicated that the primary biochemical defect in Refsum's disease lay in the conversion of phytanic acid to α-hydroxyphytanic acid, thus allowing accumulations of exogenously derived phytanic acid to occur. It therefore seems likely that Refsum's disease is due to a deficiency in phytanic acid α-hydroxylase activity. In 1966 it was reported[13] that dietary restriction of phytols and phytanates led to a fall in serum phytanic acid and some degree of clinical improvement. Malmendier et al.[14] in 1974 found that phytanic acid substituted for linoleic and arachidonic acids in the lipid sub-fractions of tissues from a patient with Refsum's disease.

Although ichthyosis has long been recognized as a component of Refsum's disease the epidermis has received little attention in this disorder. We have recently taken care of a patient with Refsum's disease in our department on whom detailed plasma and epidermal investigations have been performed.

REPORT

History

A.L. was a 37-year-old female who presented as an emergency because of extreme inanition. Her speech was unintelligible and a history was obtained from her mother. She described her daughter as being 'always frail mentally and physically'. However her early mental development appears to have been reasonably normal. She left school 'early' and subsequently led a sheltered life to be brought up by her mother.

At about 32 years of age she started developing weakness in the legs which advanced inexorably to involve the arms and rendered her bedridden for the last five months of her life. Her visual acuity progressively deteriorated during her last 6 years and scaliness of the skin became prominent during the last year of her life. She died suddenly 5 weeks after admission with a presumptive diagnosis of bronchopneumonia.

Examination

Examination revealed a grossly underweight and wasted female (Figure 8.2) with profound generalized weakness of the lower motor neurone type and a sensory peripheral neuropathy. She had incoordination of the upper limbs and

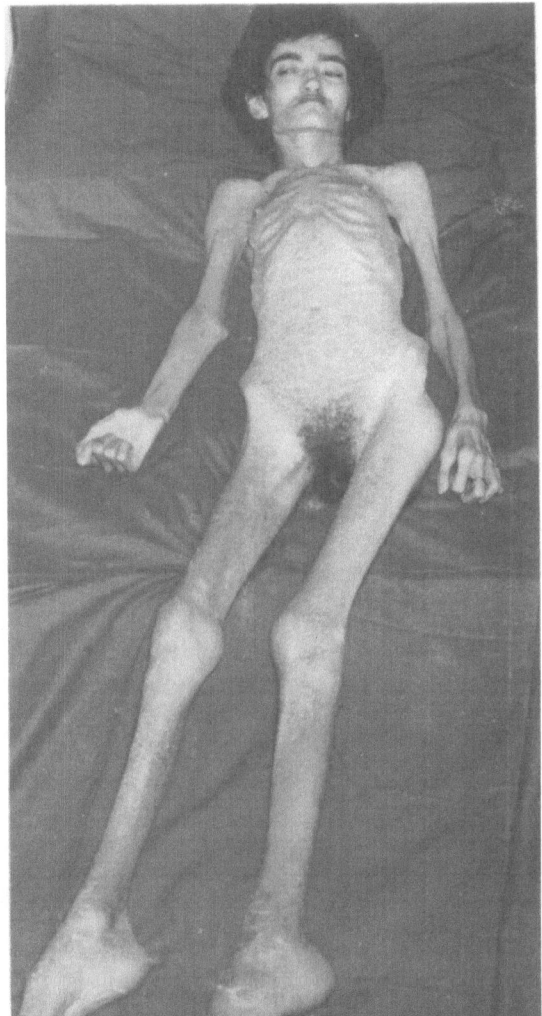

Figure 8.2 Photograph of the patient showing cachexia, gross wasting and generalized ichthyosis

pendular nystagmus. Bilateral lenticular opacities and retinitis pigmentosa were present with very poor visual acuity. There was marked generalized ichthyosis (Figure 8.3). A clinical diagnosis of Refsum's syndrome was made.

Abnormal investigations

ESR 50 mm in the first hour (Westergren); serum urea 7.9 mmol/l, K^+ 1.8 mmol/l, Cl^- 80 mmol/l and HCO_3^- 35 mmol/l; serum vitamin $B_{12} > 1000$ ng/l.

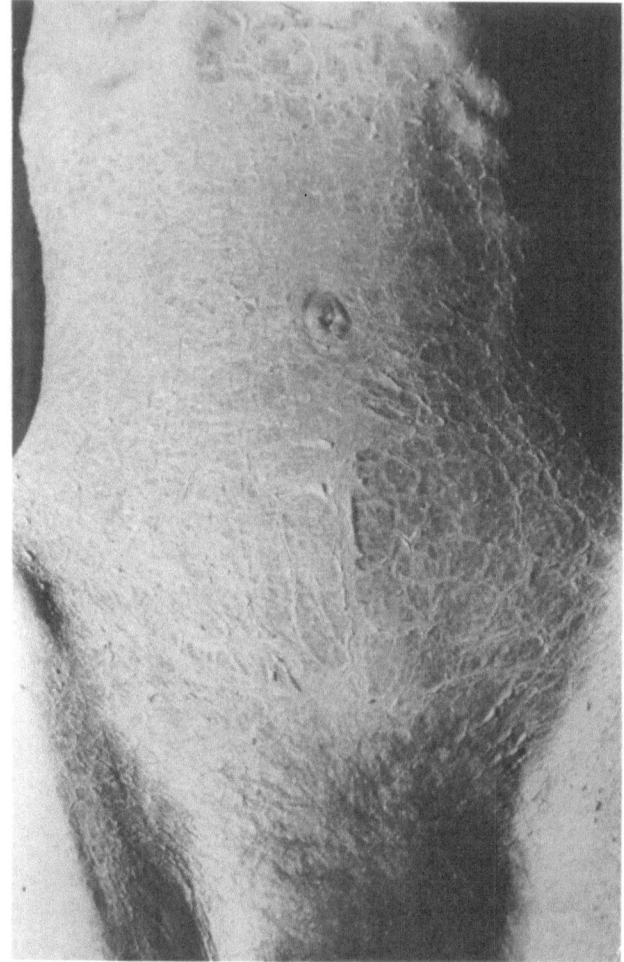

Figure 8.3   Close view of the abdomen showing the striking ichthyosis

Serum protein electrophoresis — increased α_2-globulin; serum aspartate aminotransferase 90 IU/l. The fasting plasma was turbid, triglycerides 3.8 mmol/l, lipoprotein electrophoresis — increased pre-β band; ECG. — sinus tachycardia 120/min and peaked 'P' waves. The clinical diagnosis of Refsum's disease was confirmed by the finding of large amounts of phytanic acid in the patient's plasma (vide infra).

Clinical course in hospital

Her condition in hospital remained static until about a week before death when she developed signs of a chest infection. However her condition improved only to deteriorate 48 hours before her death (6 weeks after admission).

Post-mortem findings

These were as follows:

(a) Confluent bronchopneumonia in the right lower lobe
(b) Acute tracheobronchitis
(c) Aspiration pneumonia in the left lung
(d) Fatty change in the liver and myocardium
(e) Ichthyosis.

EPIDERMAL ARCHITECTURE

Histology

Conventional light microscopy of biopsy material from the arm showed hyper-keratosis with slight acanthosis and moderate hypergranulosis but the most striking feature was the presence of vacuoles near the dermo-epidermal junction (Figure 8.4).

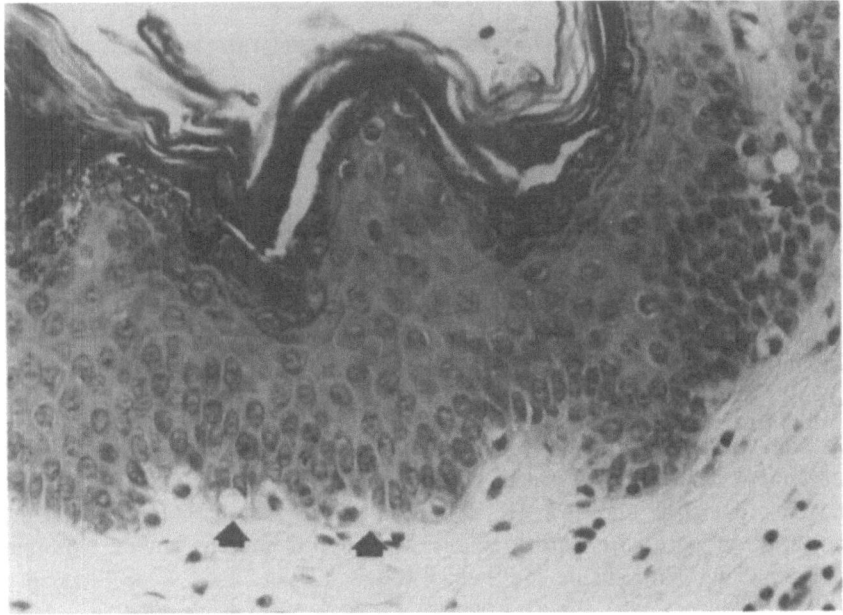

Figure 8.4 Photomicrograph of the epidermis showing vacuoles (↑) at the dermo-epidermal junction and in the basal layer of the epidermis. Moderate acanthosis, hypergranulosis and hyperkeratosis are also present. (H & E × 245)

Lipid histochemistry

Portions of skin were also quenched in a hexane/acetone CO_2 bath and subsequently cryostat-cut sections were stained for lipid using oil red O, Sudan IV and Otan staining methods[15,16]. Easily visible deposits of lipid corresponding to the vacuoles on conventional histology were demonstrated (Figure 8.5).

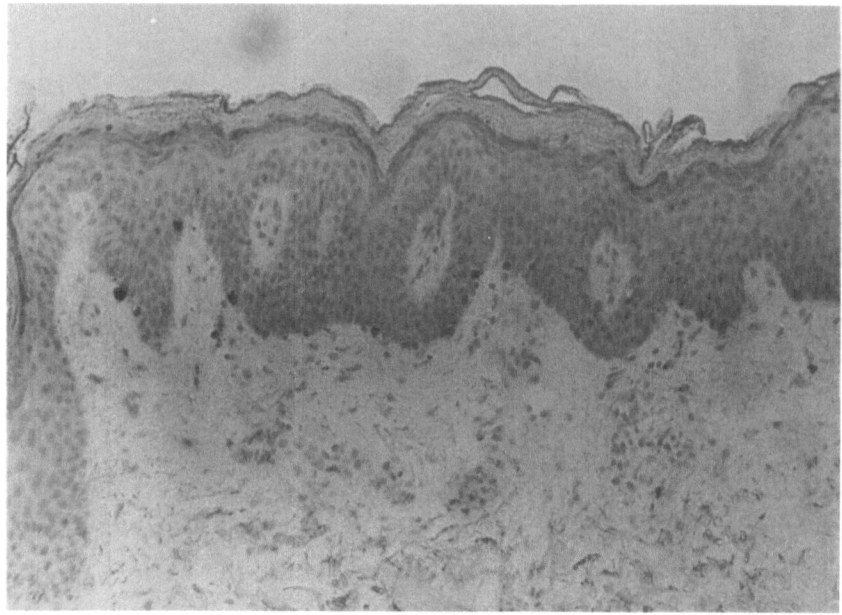

Figure 8.5 Photomicrograph of a skin biopsy stained with Otan showing lipid deposits (black) at the dermo-epidermal junction and in the basal and to a lesser extent suprabasal layers of the epidermis ($\times 105$)

Transmission Electron Microscopy

Transmission Electron Microscopy was performed on small pieces of skin fixed in 2.5% buffered glutaraldehyde, embedded in Epon and sectioned on a Leitz ultramicrotome. This revealed large vacuoles occupying an intracellular position in basal and to a lesser extent suprabasal keratinocytes of the epidermis (Figure 8.6). These vacuoles were non-membrane bound. No other abnormalities were detected in the epidermis.

Scanning Electron Microscopy

The ultrastructure of the stratum corneum was examined by scanning electron microscopy (SEM). The findings on SEM of skin surface replicas are

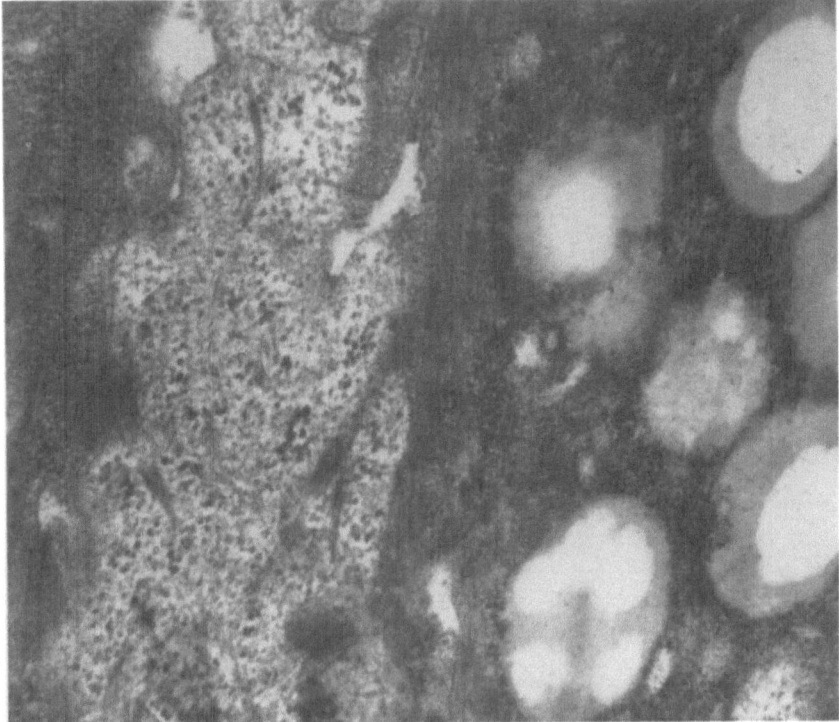

Figure 8.6 Transmission electron micrograph of basal epidermal keratinocytes showing intracellular non-membrane bound vacuoles. (×9960)

discussed elsewhere in the symposium (Chapter 12). In addition skin surface biopsies taken by the method of Marks and Dawber[17] were cut to size and stuck to aluminium stubs. They were then coated with gold in a sputter coating unit. The specimens were viewed in a Cambridge scanning electron microscope. The stratum corneum specimens showed considerable disruption in scale pattern (Figure 8.7) with large gaps easily visible between groups of corneocytes. At higher magnifications gaps were visible between individual corneocytes. The surface of individual corneocytes was somewhat irregular and showed in places small regular projections, similar but smaller than the microvillous pattern seen in psoriasis[18].

EPIDERMAL METABOLISM AND KINETICS

In vitro incorporation studies

The ^{14}C acetate *in vitro* incorporation by epidermal sheets from the patient was very high and has already been discussed in this symposium (Chapter 4). The

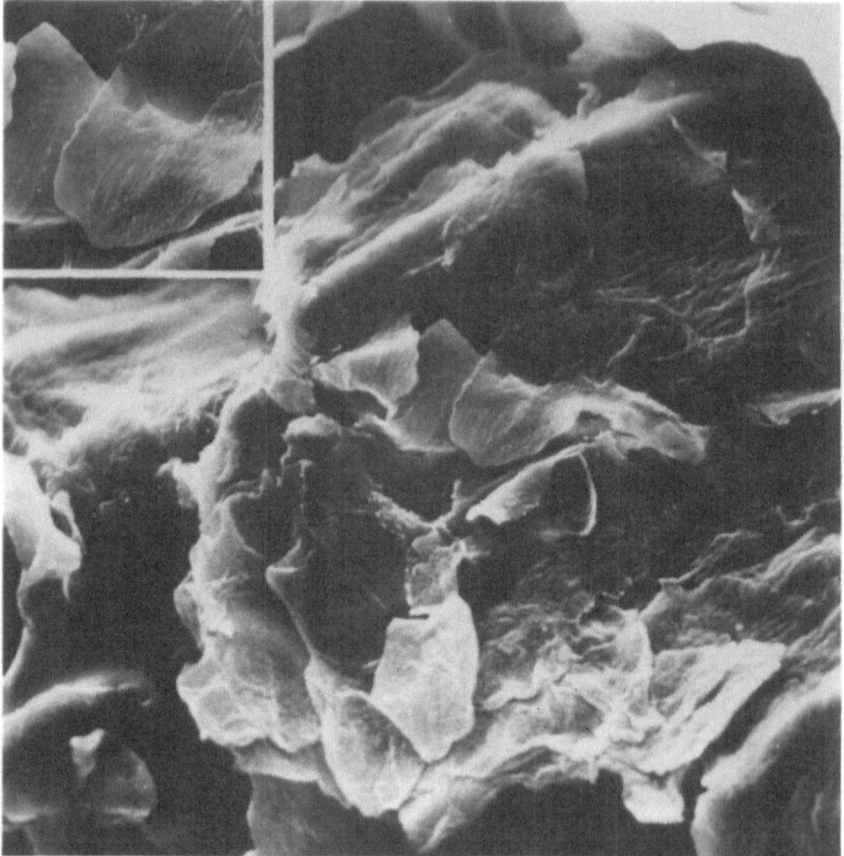

Figure 8.7 Scanning electron micrograph of a skin surface biopsy showing gross disruption in arrangement of squames with prominent gaps (×1045). Insert shows the microvillous pattern on an individual squame (×2090)

in vivo and *in vitro* labelling indices were also strikingly elevated as was the *in vitro* uptake of tritiated thymidine, proline and histidine (Chapter 6).

Enzyme histochemistry

Enzyme histochemical tests were performed on cryostat-cut frozen skin. The non-specific esterase reaction for hydrolase activity[19] showed an intense and broad band of activity in the granular cell layer and upper malpighian layer. The reactivity was much greater and more extensive than that seen in normal epidermis. Succinic dehydrogenase, lactic dehydrogenase and glucose-6-phosphate dehydrogenase reactions were also performed according to the techniques outlined by Chayen *et al.*[20] No abnormalities were detected using these techniques.

LIPID ANALYSES

Plasma

Phytanic acid content of total plasma lipid extract

Plasma lipids were extracted by the method of Folch *et al.*[21] after the addition of an internal standard. Standards of phytanic acid were similarly treated. Constituent fatty acids were then converted to their methyl esters and analysed by gas–liquid chromatography. The phytanic acid content was calculated by comparison of the ratio of the peak heights of phytanate to internal standard for the test with those for the standard. Phytanic acid was also calculated as a percentage of all fatty acids from C_{14} to C_{20} by comparison of peak areas calculated from the product of peak height and retention time. The results are shown in Table 8.1 where it can be seen that phytanic acid accounts for 50% of the total plasma fatty acids.

Table 8.1   Peak identification and percentage of total serum fatty acids

Myristic acid	(14:0)	0.5%
Internal standard		
Palmitic acid	(16:0)	13%
Palmitoleic acid	(16:1)	1.1%
Phytanic acid	(br–20:0)	50%
Stearic acid	(18:0)	1.7%
Oleic acid	(18:1)	16%
Linoleic acid	(18:2)	9.1%
Unknown peak (not normally present)		1.6%
Linolenic acid	(18:3)	0.4%
Unknown peak (normally present)		0.6%
Position of 5,8,11-eicosatrienoic acid $(20:3\omega9)$		0%
8,11,14-eicosatrienoic acid $(20:3\omega6)$		0.3%
Arachidonic acid $(20:4\omega6)$		5.0%

Phytanic acid content of plasma lipid subfractions

Plasma lipids were extracted using a modification of the method of Folch *et al.*[21] After concentration, the lipid extract was quantitatively analysed by silica gel thin layer chromatography. The patient's plasma was analysed in duplicate with a normal plasma for comparison as shown in Figure 8.8. The most striking feature is the large amount of triglyceride present in the patient with Refsum's disease which is in three parts. Individual spots were then quantitatively extracted, transmethylated and analysed by gas–liquid chromatography for phytanic acid. The results are shown in Table 8.2 as percentages of phytanic in the lipid subfractions. It can be seen that phytanic acid accounts for 48% of the total fatty acid, agreeing well with the figure of 50% obtained by gas–liquid chromatography of the total lipid extract (Table 8.1). Phytanic acid is found in all lipid subfractions particularly triglycerides

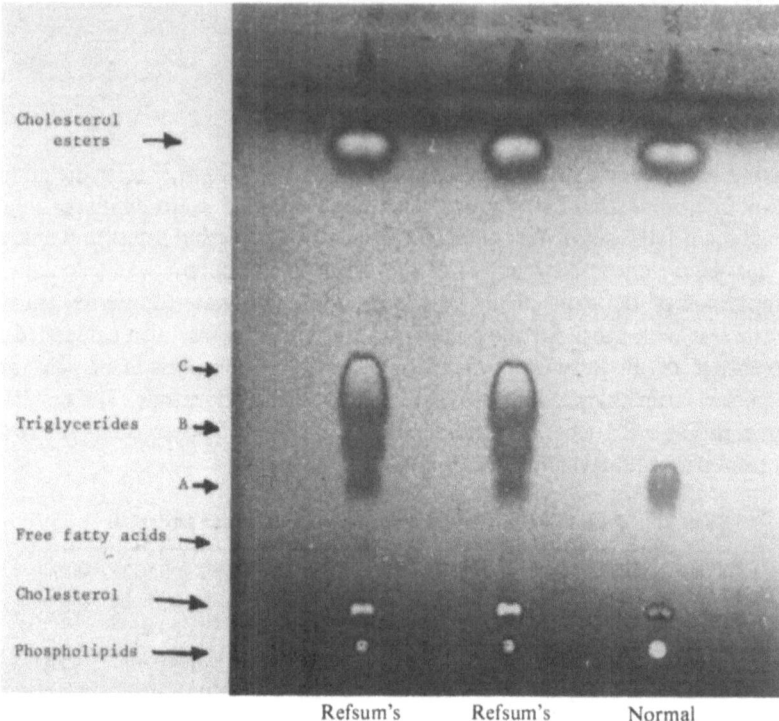

Refsum's   Refsum's   Normal

Figure 8.8 Thin layer chromatography of plasma lipid extracts from the patient (left-hand and middle 'runs') and from a normal control (right-hand 'run')

and phospholipids. It is of interest that whereas the slow-moving 'normal' triglyceride fraction contains only 8% of phytanic acid, the intermediate (B) and fast (C) moving fractions contain 47% and 74% of phytanic acid respectively. In (B) one and in (C) two of the fatty acids esterified to glycerol are phytanic acid[22].

Table 8.2 Distribution of phytanic acid in plasma

Lipid fraction	Concentration of phytanate (mg/ml plasma)	Phytanate as % of fatty acids C_{14} to C_{20}
Total	3.10	48
Cholesterol esters	0.05	4.5
Triglycerides		
fast moving fraction	1.80	74
intermediate fraction	0.25	47
slow moving fraction	0.01	8
Free fatty acids	0.02	25
Phospholipids	1.13	46

Epidermis

A sheet of skin from one thigh of the patient was obtained by keratotome biopsy (Castroviejo keratotome set at 0.4 mm). Epidermis was prepared from this by heating in saline at 60 °C for 4 minutes. After freeze-drying and desiccation, the samples were weighed and analysed as described for the plasma. Samples of skin from two normal subjects were prepared and analysed in an identical way for comparison. The percentage of phytanic acid in the epidermal lipid subfractions is shown in Table 8.3. Large amounts of phytanic acid were found in all subfractions. Each subfraction was then analysed for individual fatty acid content and the results are shown in Table 8.4.

Table 8.3 Phytanic acid content of lipid sub-fractions of epidermis

Fraction	Wt. of phytanate μg/mg dry weight	Phytanate expressed as % of total fatty acid C_{14}–C_{20} in the fraction
Phospholipids	8.4	45
Free fatty acids	1.9	20
Triglycerides	5.3	72
Cholesterol esters	1.7	35

Sebum

Sebum from the patient was obtained using the method of Cunliffe and Shuster[23]. The extracted lipids (total) were analysed for fatty acid content by gas–liquid chromatography and the results are shown in Table 8.5. From this limited data it can be seen that phytanic acid seems to be incorporated into sebum lipids, although possible contamination from epidermal lipids cannot be excluded.

DISCUSSION

Our studies (light microscopy and TEM) have shown the presence of morphologically visible lipid deposits in the basal layer of the epidermis in this patient with Refsum's Disease. In a transmission electron microscopy study Anton-Lamprecht and Kahlke[24] have similarly demonstrated the presence of intracellular 'liposomes' in the lower part of the epidermis. They also found (in contrast to our findings) a reduction in the epidermal granular cell layer to one cell thickness and decreased amounts of keratohyalin. In addition their study showed retardation in the dissolution of desmosomal discs which began around the twenty-fifth horn cell layer. Our patient showed hypergranulosis and a strikingly increased non-specific esterase activity in the upper epidermis. The results of kinetic and other metabolic studies showed markedly increased epidermopoiesis and metabolic activity. SEM performed on skin surface biopsies showed a profound disruption in overall scale pattern and at higher

Table 8.4   Fatty acid composition of epidermal lipid subfractions

	Normal 1		Normal 2		Refsum's	
	(% of FAs C_{14} to C_{20})	(µg/mg dry wt.)	(% of FAs C_{14} to C_{20})	(µg/mg dry wt.)	(% of FAs C_{14} to C_{20})	(µg/mg dry wt.)
Phospholipid						
14:0	0.8	0.11	0.7	0.1	1.3	0.24
16:0	15.0	2.03	15.5	2.43	15.0	2.84
16:1	1.1	0.15	1.3	0.2	1.7	0.31
Phytanic	0	0	0	0	45.0	8.39
18:0	12.5	1.69	13.2	2.07	6.2	1.14
18:1	17.5	2.37	18.5	2.89	13.0	2.45
18:2	37.0	5.01	36.2	5.65	5.4	1.0
18:3	0.5	0.07	0.7	0.11	0.4	0.08
20:3ω6	2.1	0.28	1.7	0.26	2.6	0.47
20:4ω6	5.8	0.78	5.4	0.84	2.6	0.49
Free fatty acids						
14:0	3.4	0.07	3.7	0.1	2.2	0.2
16:0	22.3	0.45	21.9	0.57	10.0	1.91
16:1	2.9	0.06	3.4	0.09	1.6	0.15
Phytanic	0	0	0	0	20.0	1.9
18:0	13.6	0.28	17.0	0.44	20.0	1.85
18:1	11.8	0.24	19.5	0.51	19.0	1.76
18:2	18.2	0.37	16.4	0.43	5.6	0.53
18:3	0.6	0.01	0.7	0.02	0.6	0.06
20:3ω6	0.8	0.02	0.6	0.02	0	0
20:4ω6	18.1	0.37	11.7	0.31	8.0	0.76
Triglycerides						
14:0	5.6	0.07	6.9	0.08	1.3	0.1
16:0	27.2	0.33	26.3	0.32	11.0	0.84
16:1	10.2	0.12	11.3	0.14	0.9	0.07
Phytanic	0	0	0	0	72.0	5.3
18:0	9.3	0.11	12.2	0.15	3.1	0.22
18:1	29.9	0.37	25.9	0.31	7.5	0.55
18:2	11.4	0.14	7.5	0.09	1.2	0.09
18:3	1.0	0.01	1.8	0.02	0.4	0.03
20:3ω6	1.3	0.02	2.2	0.03	0.3	0.02
20:4ω6	0.6	0.01	1.5	0.02	0.6	0.04
Cholesterol esters						
14:0	2.3	0.04	2.5	0.04	3.0	0.15
16:0	9.5	0.15	11.0	0.2	23.0	1.1
16:1	9.0	0.14	8.9	0.16	2.5	0.12
Phytanic	0	0	0	0	35.0	1.7
18:0	3.0	0.05	3.9	0.07	7.4	0.36
18:1	53.0	0.86	50.5	0.92	17.0	0.84
18:2	16.9	0.27	15.8	0.29	7.4	0.36
18:3	0.8	0.01	0.9	0.02	1.3	0.06
20:3ω6	0.8	0.01	1.0	0.02	0.8	0.04
20:4ω6	2.0	0.03	2.5	0.05	2.2	0.11

magnification, the suggestion of a microvillous pattern on individual corneo-cytes. This latter finding is often seen in scaling conditions characterized by 'high output' epidermopoiesis[18], which our patient certainly had.

Table 8.5   Fatty acid composition of sebum

Fatty acid	Percentage of total FA
$C_{14}:0$	10
$C_{16}:0$	29
$C_{16}:1$	30
Phytanate	4
$C_{18}:0$	11
$C_{18}:1$	15

The biochemical analyses have revealed considerable quantities of free and esterified phytanic acid in plasma and epidermis. In the latter, large amounts of phytanic acid was found in all lipid subfractions. Analysis of the phospholipid subfraction in this patient and of two normal controls (Table 8.4) showed a striking reduction in linoleic acid (18:2) content from a mean of 36.6% in the controls to 5.4% in the patient with Refsum's disease. A similar, though less marked reduction was observed in the arachidonic acid (20:4 ω6) levels in the epidermal phospholipid subfraction in the patient with Refsum's disease. Both linoleic acid and arachidonic acid are known to be essential fatty acids in man and animals[25] a deficiency producing an ichthyosis-like scaling dermatosis.

It would appear that in Refsum's disease the epidermis (as with other tissues) substitutes phytanic acid for essential fatty acids in all lipid subfractions and especially phospholipid. This is most likely a reflection of the large amounts of phytanic acid present in fatty acid intra- and extracellular pools. On the basis of the above it is suggested that the abnormal epidermal findings in Refsum's disease result from the incorporation of phytanic acid into epidermal lipids with failure in their degradation. Evidence for a failure in degradation comes from the work of Laurell[26] who found that plasma post-heparin lipase was incapable of splitting glyceryl triphytanate whereas glyceryl tripalmitate was easily hydrolysed.

It is of interest that in both EFA deficiency and Refsum's syndrome there is an altered phospholipid profile and in contrast with other 'non-erythematous' ichthyotic states there is a marked elevation of epidermopoiesis. All membranes contain much phospholipid. The above observation and the well-known localization of 5-nucleotidase activity in the plasma membrane might suggest a particular relationship between this structure and mitotic activity.

References

1. Refsum, S. (1946). Heredopathia atactica polyneuritiformis. *Acta Psychiatr. Scand.*, **38**, (Suppl) 1
2. Klenk, E. and Kahlke, W. (1963). Uber das Vorkommen der 3,7,11,15-tetra-methylhexadecansäure (phytansäure) in den cholesterinestern und anderen lipoidfraktionen der organe bei einem krankheitsfall unbekannter genese (verdacht auf heredopathia atactica polyneuritiformis (Refsum-Syndrom). *Hoppe Seyler Z. Physiol. Chem.*, **333**, 133
3. Kahlke, W. (1964). Refsum-Syndrom. Lipoidchemische Untersuchungen bei 9 Fällen. *Klin. Wochenschr.*, **42**, 1011

4. Avigan, J. (1966). The presence of phytanic acid in normal human and animal plasma. *Biochim. Biophys. Acta*, **116,** 391

5. Steinberg, D., Avigan, J., Mize, C., Eldjarn, L., Try, L. and Refsum, S. (1965). Conversion of U-C^{14} phytol to phytanic acid and its oxidation in heredopathia atactica polyneuritiformis. *Biochem. Biophys. Res. Comm.*, **19,** 783

6. Steinberg, D., Mize, C. E., Avigan, J., Fales, H. M., Eldjarn, L., Try, K., Stokke, O. and Refsum, S. (1966). Studies on the metabolic error in Refsum's disease. *J. Clin. Invest.*, **45,** 1076

7. Steinberg, D., Mize, C. E., Avigan, J., Fales, H. M., Eldjarn, L., Try, K., Stokke, O. and Refsum, S. (1967). Studies on the metabolic error in Refsum's disease. *J. Clin. Invest.*, **46,** 313

8. Steinberg, D., Avigan, J., Mize, C. E., Baxter, J. H., Cammermeyer, J., Fales, H. M. and Highet, P. F. (1966). Effects of dietary phytols and phytanic acid in animals. *J. Lipid Res.*, **7,** 684

9. Steinberg, D. (1972). Phytanic acid storage disease. Refsum's syndrome. In, *The Metabolic Basis of Inherited Disease*. J. B. Stanbury, J. B. Wyngaarden and D. S. Fredrickson (eds.). 3rd Ed. pp. 833–853 (New York: McGraw-Hill)

10. Steinberg, D., Herndon, J. H., Uhlendorf, B. W., Mize, C. E., Avigan, J. and Milne, G. W. A. (1967). Refsum's disease. Nature of the enzyme defect. *Science*, **156,** 1740.

11. Steinberg, D., Avigan, J., Mize, C. E., Herndon, J. H., Fales, H. M. and Milne, G. W. A. (1968). The nature of the metabolic defect in Refsum's disease. *Path Eur.*, **3,** 450

12. Herndon, J. H., Steinberg, D., Uhlendorft, B. W. and Fales, H. M. (1969). Refsum's disease: characterization of the enzyme defect in cell culture. *J. Clin. Invest.*, **48,** 1017

13. Eldjarn, L., Try, K., Stokke, O., Munthe-Kaas, A. W., Refsum, S., Steinberg, D., Avigan, J. and Mize, C. (1966). Dietary effects on serum phytanic acid levels and on clinical manifestations in heredopathia atactica polyneuritiformis. *Lancet*, **1,** 691

14. Malmendier, C. L., Jonniaux, G., Voet, W. and Van den Bergen, C. J. (1974). Fatty acid composition of tissues in Refsum's disease (heredopathia atactica polyneuritiformis). Estimation of total phytanic acid accumulation. *Biomedicine*, **20,** 398

15. Chayen, J., Bitensky, L. and Butcher, R. (1973). Practical Histochemistry, pp. 81–83 (London: John Wiley and Sons)

16. Pearse, A. G. E. (1968). *Histochemistry Theoretical and Applied.* 3rd Ed. Vol 1, p. 694 (J. and A. Churchill Ltd)

17. Marks, R. and Dawber, R. P. R. (1971). Skin surface biopsy. An improved technique for examination of the stratum corneum. *Br. J. Dermatol.*, **84,** 117

18. Griffiths, W. A. D. and Marks, R. (1973). The significance of surface changes in parakeratotic horn. *J. Invest. Dermatol.*, **61,** 251

19. Holt, S. J. (1952). A new principle for the histochemical localization of hydrolytic enzymes. *Nature (London)*, **169,** 271

20. Chayen, J., Bitensky, L. and Butcher, R. (1973). *Practical Histochemistry* (London: John Wiley & Sons)

21. Folch, J., Lees, M. and Sloane-Stanley, G. H. (1957). A simple method for the isolation and purification of total lipids from animal tissues. *J. Biol. Chem.*, **226,** 497

22. Karlsson, K. A., Norrby, A. and Samuelsson, B. (1967). Use of thin layer chromatography for the preliminary diagnosis of Refsum's disease (Heredopathia atactica polyneuritiformis). *Biochim. Biophys. Acta*, **144,** 162

23. Cunliffe, W. J. and Shuster, S. (1969). The rate of sebum secretion in man. *Br. J. Dermatol.*, **81,** 697

24. Anton-Lamprecht, L. and Kahlke, W. (1974). Zur Ultrastruktur hereditarer Verhornungsstörungen. V. Ichthyosis bein Refsum-Syndrom (Heredopathia atactica polyneuritiformis). *Arch. Dermatol. Forsch.*, **250,** 185

25. Prottey, C. (1976). Essential fatty acid and the skin. *Br. J. Dermatol.*, **94,** 579

26. Laurell, S. (1958). The action of lipoprotein lipase on glyceryl triphytanate. *Biochim. Biophys. Acta*, **152,** 80

9
Ultrastructural Features of Ichthyotic Skin in Refsum's Syndrome

CL. BLANCHET-BARDON, I. ANTON-LAMPRECHT, A. PUISSANT and U. W. SCHNYDER

INTRODUCTION

We wish to report two cases of Refsum's syndrome, the first coming from the University of Heidelberg, the second from the Dermatology Department of Paris (Professeur Duperrat, Professeur Puissant). Both cases developed ichthyosis and have been investigated for epidermal ultrastructural changes. In the second case, a further biopsy was available after 4 years of a chlorophyll-free diet.

Refsum's syndrome is inherited as an autosomal recessive trait. It is characterized by an enzymatic defect of α-oxidation resulting in an accumulation of phytanic acid in many organs and body fluids. This fatty acid is a result of incomplete degradation of phytol, a part of the chlorophyll molecule.

The main features and their incidence in a total of 44 cases were documented by Kahlke[1]. Skin changes are present in about 54% of all patients. They are reported to be related to the degree of phytanic acid storage and to disappear with treatment.

THE PATIENTS AND METHODS

The diagnosis of Refsum's syndrome in our patients was made — on the clinical features which had developed progressively over many years since early adolescence — and biochemically by the high level of phytanic acid in the blood — 20% of the serum fatty acids, in case 1 and 26% in case 2. Both cases show all the clinical features of the disease. In the second case yellow naevi appeared on the trunk and the limbs, and a phytanic acid assay of these lesions showed 1.9 μg per mg of tissue.

The histological findings were the same in both cases. The basal layer of the epidermis contained cells with large cytoplasmic vacuoles regularly distributed every 3 to 6 cells. The disposition of these cells suggested that they could be epidermal melanocytes. The granular layer was reduced to a single cell layer. There was also hyperkeratosis. In the dermal naevus the melanocytes of the superficial half are globular and distorted by vacuoles which completely fill the cytoplasm and push the nucleus to the periphery of the cell. On frozen sections, oil red O intensively stained the content of the cytoplasmic vacuoles, both in the epidermis and in the naevus.

Ultrastructurally in the second case the dermal naevus cells contained numerous mitochondria in close proximity to the cytoplasmic vacuoles. The ultrastructural findings in the epidermis were the same in both cases

Quantitative deviations in the granular and horny layer resulted in moderate hyperkeratosis. The granular layer was reduced to a single layer with a decrease of keratohyalin, which was, however, structurally normal (Figure 9.1). Keratinosomes were found in normal numbers. The horny layer was 30 to

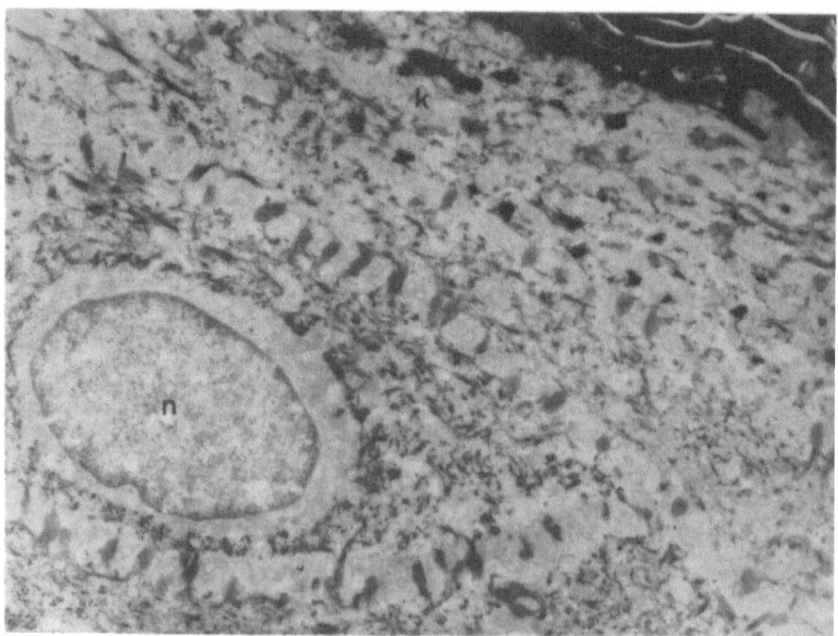

Figure 9.1 A single cellular layer with decrease of keratohyalin which is structurally normal (×6700)

40 cells thick and showed in part a typical keratin pattern. The dissolution of desmosomal discs was obviously retarded and began around the 25th horn cell layer. No structural abnormalities were found in desmosomes, tonofibrils or keratinosomes.

In the lower epidermal strata lipid droplets were present in the cytoplasm of keratinocytes and melanocytes (Figure 9.2). In the cytoplasm of the basal and

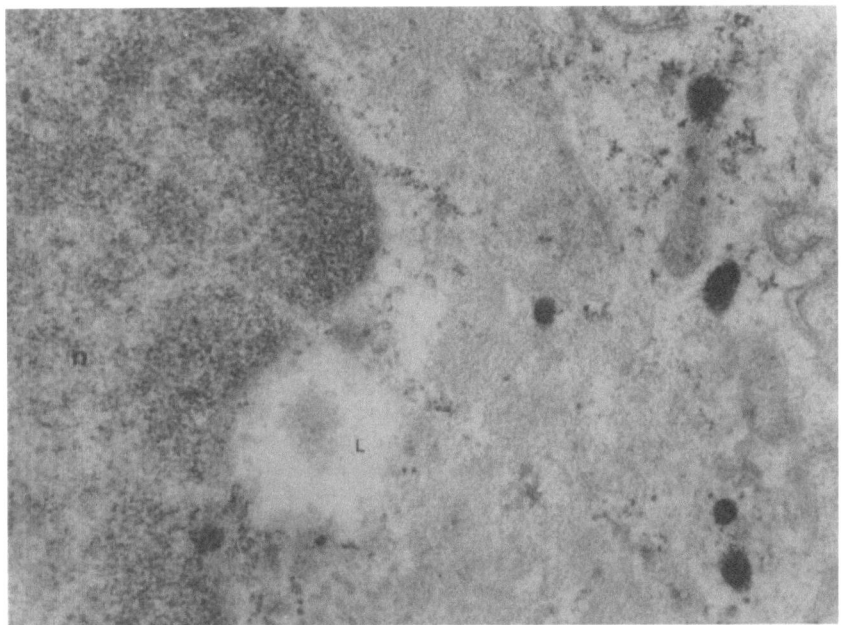

Figure 9.2   Lipid droplet (L) in the cytoplasm of basal cell (×40 200)

prickle cells the vacuoles were found amongst tonofibrils, mitochondria and melanosome complexes. The lipid droplets also showed a close proximity to endoplasmic reticulum and abnormal or giant mitochondria. These giant degenerate mitochondria had a poorly developed internal membrane system and a matrix of poor contrast and increased amounts of DNA. Since these vacuoles were largely depleted of fat after extraction it may indicate that they are composed of neutral fats and saturated fatty acids and might therefore represent phytanic acid esterified with cholesterol or triglyceride.

After 4 years treatment on a chlorophyll-free diet, the second patient showed clinical improvement with a decrease in ichthyosis. The epidermis had a granular layer 3–4 cells thick. In the basal layer there were lipid droplets and the oil red O stain was negative. Ultrastructurally the granular layer had three cell layers with slightly decreased amounts of keratohyalin which is structurally normal. The stratum corneum consisted of 20 to 25 flat horny cells (Figure 9.3). In the lower epidermis few liposomes were present in the keratinocytes.

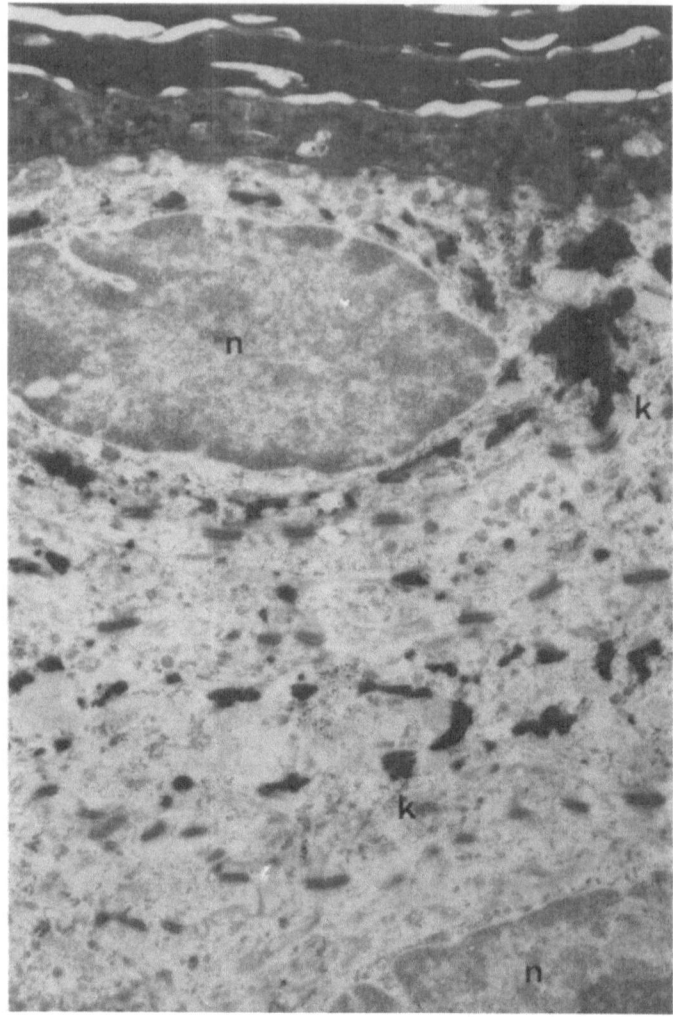

Figure 9.3 Ultrastructural situation in the granular layer after dietary treatment (×12 000)

The melanocytes contained more lipid droplets than the keratinocytes and these droplets were again in proximity to giant and abnormal mitochondria (Figure 9.4).

Thus after 4 years treatment the accumulation of lipids was decreased in keratinocytes but less so in melanocytes. It would appear that the melanocytes are more sensitive to the high phytanic acid level than the keratinocytes.

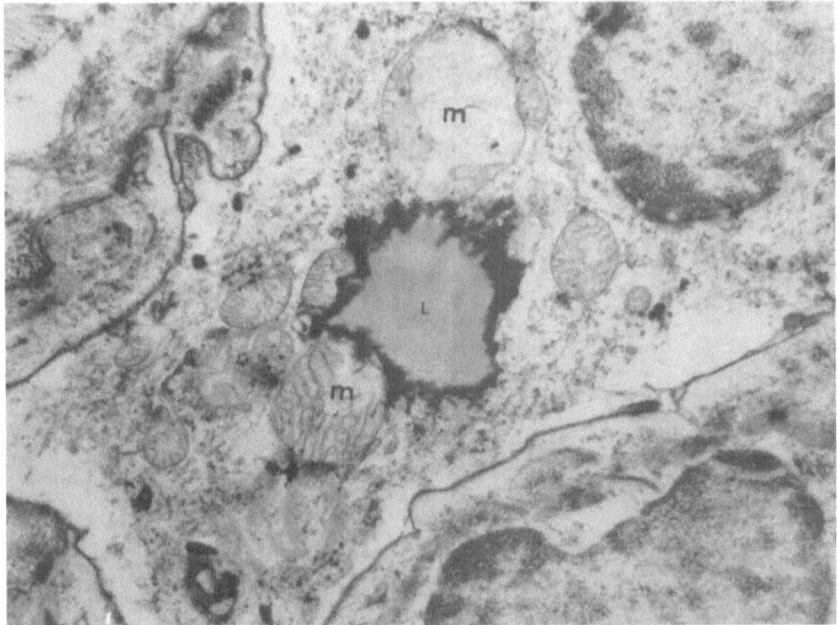

Figure 9.4 Persistence in the melanocytes of lipid droplet (*L*) in proximity to giant and abnormal mitochondria (*M*) (×20 100)

CONCLUSIONS

We therefore suggest the following hypothesis on the correlation of ichthyosiform skin changes and disturbed lipid metabolism in Refsum's syndrome. High amounts of phytanic acid accumulate due to a gene-dependent enzymatic defect in α-oxidation. Free cholesterol is esterified by phytanic acid and phytanic acid-bound cholesterol is subsequently stored in the epidermal liposome. This leads to a decrease of free epidermal cholesterol and results in disturbances of normal keratinization. The beneficial results of 4 years of chlorophyll-free diet support this hypothesis.

References

1. Kahlke, W. (1967). Heredopathia atactica polyneuritiformis (Refsum's Disease). In G. Schettler (ed.) *Lipids and Lipidoses* (Berlin, Heidelberg, New York: Springer)

10
Ultrastructural Criteria for the Distinction of Different Types of Inherited Ichthyoses

I. ANTON-LAMPRECHT

SUMMARY

Electron microscopic studies in different types of inherited ichthyoses have been used as a basis for classifying this large group of 'inborn errors of keratinization'. Ultrastructural abnormalities of structural proteins such as keratohyalin and tonofilaments have been shown to be an intrinsic feature of some dominantly inherited types (keratohyalin defect in autosomal dominant ichthyosis vulgaris, disturbances of tonofibrillar distribution in bullous ichthyosiform erythroderma or ichthyosis hystrix type Curth–Macklin), whereas only quantitative deviations from the normal keratinization process occur in recessively transmitted types (X-linked recessive ichthyosis Wells–Kerr, lamellar ichthyosis). Ultrastructural criteria may thus well serve as parameters for diagnosis in doubtful cases. Moreover, the ichthyoses provide a suitable model system for an analysis of the keratinization process and of the mode of gene interaction during this sequence of differentiative steps of keratinizing cells.

INTRODUCTION

Ultrastructural studies in inherited ichthyoses were primarily performed in order to provide criteria for a better classification of this heterogeneous group of genodermatoses. However, it turns out that the ichthyoses as the most important group of 'inborn errors of keratinization' may well serve as a

71

model system for an analysis of the keratinization process and for our understanding of how genes interact in this process[1].

For the classification of genodermatoses four main parameters are at present available; these are (1) clinical features, (2) genetics, (3) histopathology, and (4) ultrastructural criteria. Presumably biochemical data will be included in the future. Based on the above parameters, the inherited ichthyoses may at present be classified according to the following groups[2,3]:

—ichthyosis vulgaris group
—ichthyosis congenita group (lamellar ichthyosis)
—hystrix-like ichthyoses

Following this rough classification, some ultrastructural criteria will be presented for the most important types of ichthyoses, even though it is not possible to fully describe the entire keratinization process for each of them. Only those parameters that may serve as diagnostic aids will be discussed.

As a basis for a better understanding of the following presentation the ultra-structural features of the process of keratinization will briefly be mentioned.

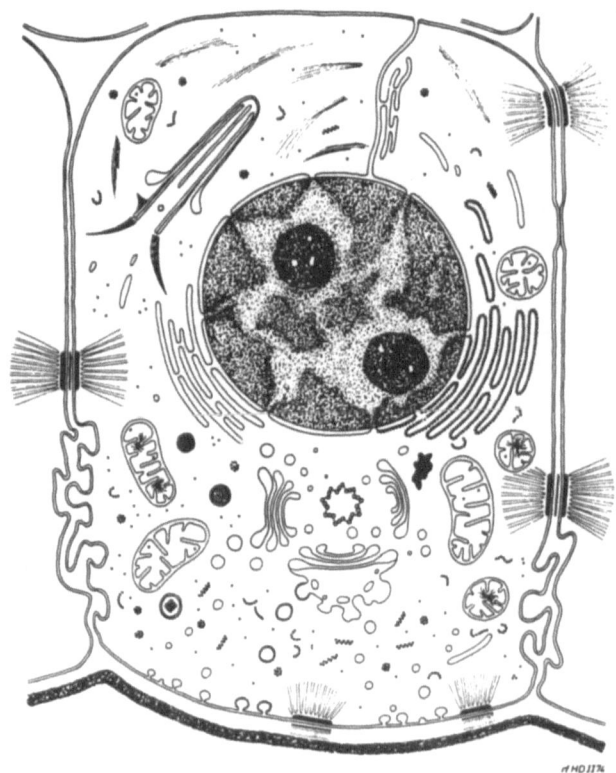

Figure 10.1 Schematic representation of the ultrastructural organization of a normal epidermal basal cell

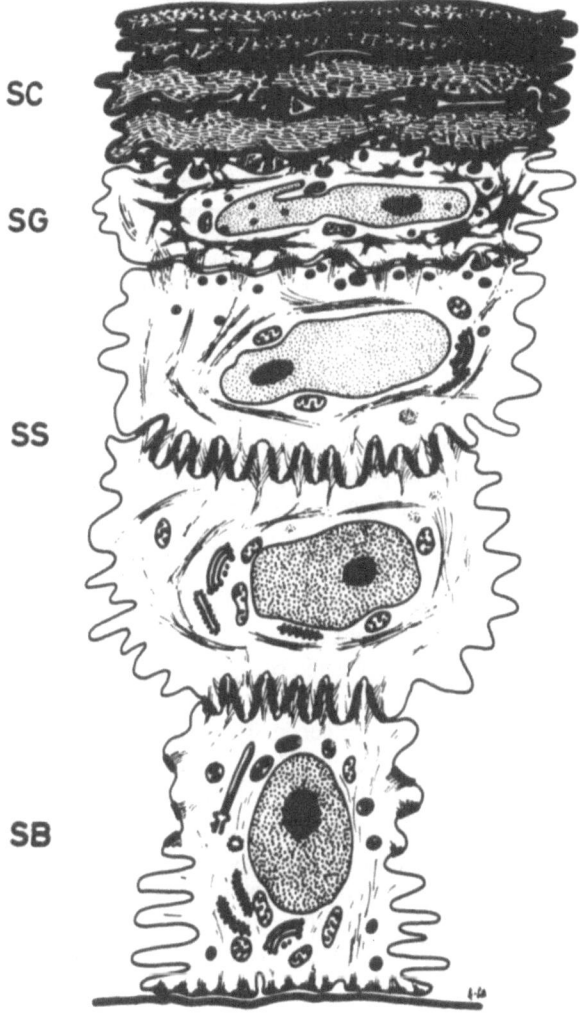

Figure 10.2 Schematic drawing of an epidermal cell column summing up the differentiative and synthetic steps of the keratinization process. SB — stratum basale, SS — stratum spinosum, SG — stratum granulosum, SC — stratum corneum. (From: Anton-Lamprecht and Schnyder[1], with kind permission of Springer Verlag Heidelberg)

Epidermal cells show all normal cellular structures including nucleus, mitochondria, Golgi bodies, endoplasmic reticulum, lysosomes, polyribosomes, and plasma membrane, as well as some structural specializations that are typical elements of ectodermal tissues: e.g. desmosomes, and tonofilaments (Figure 10.1). During the normal keratinization process, cells move up singly, passing through a sequence of differentiative and synthetic steps (Figure 10.2).

Table 10.1

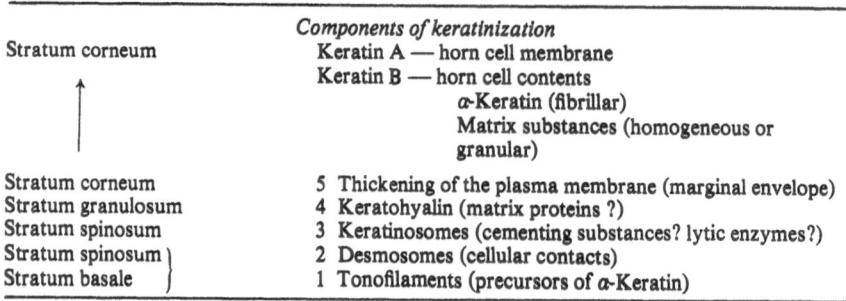

	Components of keratinization
Stratum corneum	Keratin A — horn cell membrane
	Keratin B — horn cell contents
	α-Keratin (fibrillar)
	Matrix substances (homogeneous or granular)
Stratum corneum	5 Thickening of the plasma membrane (marginal envelope)
Stratum granulosum	4 Keratohyalin (matrix proteins ?)
Stratum spinosum	3 Keratinosomes (cementing substances? lytic enzymes?)
Stratum spinosum	2 Desmosomes (cellular contacts)
Stratum basale	1 Tonofilaments (precursors of α-Keratin)

Five components are typical products of keratinizing epidermal cells (Table 10.1); tonofilaments and desmosomes are formed in increasing amounts in the prickle cell layer, tonofilaments being precursors of the α-keratin fibrils of horn cells. In the upper Malpighian layers keratinosomes (or Odland bodies) are formed; they discharge their contents to the intercellular spaces where they appear to constitute cementing substances and thus seem to be in the main part responsible for the barrier function of the epidermis[4]. Keratohyalin is synthesized as the next step in the granular layer. Its proteins appear to contribute to matrix substances of the horny cells together with remnants of the breakdown of nuclear and cytoplasmic components. Just before cells enter into the horny layer, the marginal envelope is formed by an apposition of proteinaceous substances to the inner leaflet of the plasma membrane, which incidentally isolates the cell from its physiological (and nutritional) environment. The horn cells with their highly resistant membranes and their contents of α-keratin fibrils and matrix substances are the end product of this sequence of differentiative and synthetic steps.

Disturbances may occur in each of these stages, induced either by environmental factors or — in the case of the ichthyoses — by mutation of different genes. In many types the resulting 'error in keratinization' is directly demonstrable in the ultrastructural deviations from the normal keratinization process.

ICHTHYOSIS VULGARIS GROUP

In *X-linked ichthyosis* the granular layer is always present, as Wells and others[5-9] have shown, though sometimes reduced or, in other cases, increased, as compared to normal skin, and keratohyalin granules are always demonstrable. On the other hand, in *autosomal dominant ichthyosis vulgaris*, clinically often represented only by follicular keratosis and very mild scaling, a granular layer is almost completely missing by light and electron microscopy. Only single cells below the horny layer reveal a low amount of granular

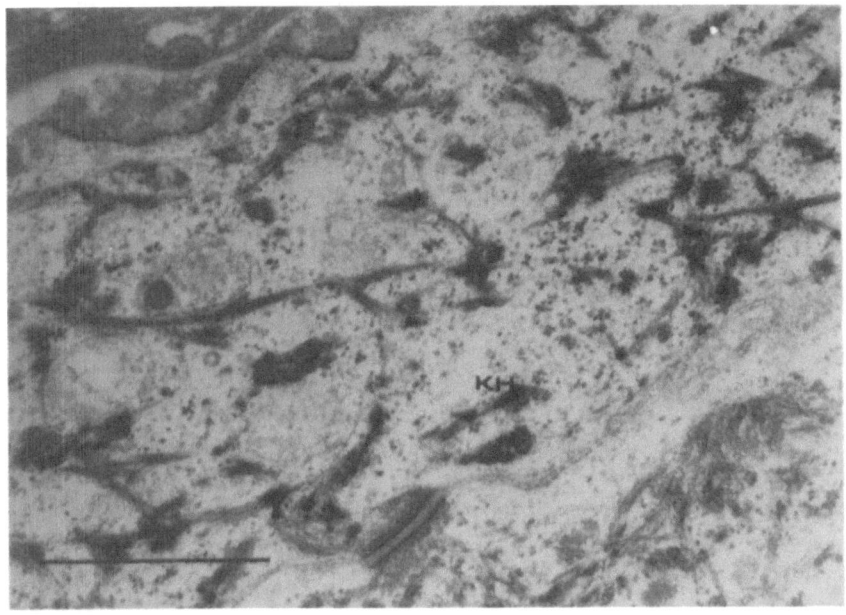

a

b

Figure 10.3   Comparison of keratohyalin (KH) amount and ultrastructure in autosomal dominant ichthyosis vulgaris (a) and X-linked recessive ichthyosis (b); ×31 500

components. At higher magnifications the intrinsic difference between both types of ichthyosis is revealed as the defective keratohyalin synthesis in the dominant type (Figure 10.3). In X-linked ichthyosis large amounts of a normally structured keratohyalin are formed[10], whereas in dominant ichthyosis only small amounts of abnormal keratohyalin granules of 'crumbly' appearance are synthesized. This abnormal keratohyalin is a constant feature of autosomal dominant ichthyosis vulgaris (ADI)[11,12] and represents a structural defect of a structural protein. The same abnormal keratohyalin ultrastructure is present in those cases in whom ADI is combined with an atopic diathesis. In X-linked ichthyosis (XRI) transitional cells are more easily found than in all other types of ichthyosis[10]. They may also serve as a diagnostic criterion in doubtful cases.

Refsum's syndrome will only briefly be mentioned here, since our studies together with the dermatologic department of Professor Duperrat and Professor Puissant are reported by Dr. Blanchet-Bardon in more detail (Chapter 9). Though very similar to autosomal dominant ichthyosis vulgaris histopathologically, ichthyosis in Refsum's syndrome may be strictly differentiated from the dominant type by the consistently normal keratohyalin ultrastructure[13].

No significant deviations of mitotic rate and turnover time have up to now been found according to Frost[14,15] in the group of vulgar ichthyoses. They are characterized by a retention hyperkeratosis (Schnyder[16]). This may at least in part be due to the late dissolution of the desmosomal plates in the horny

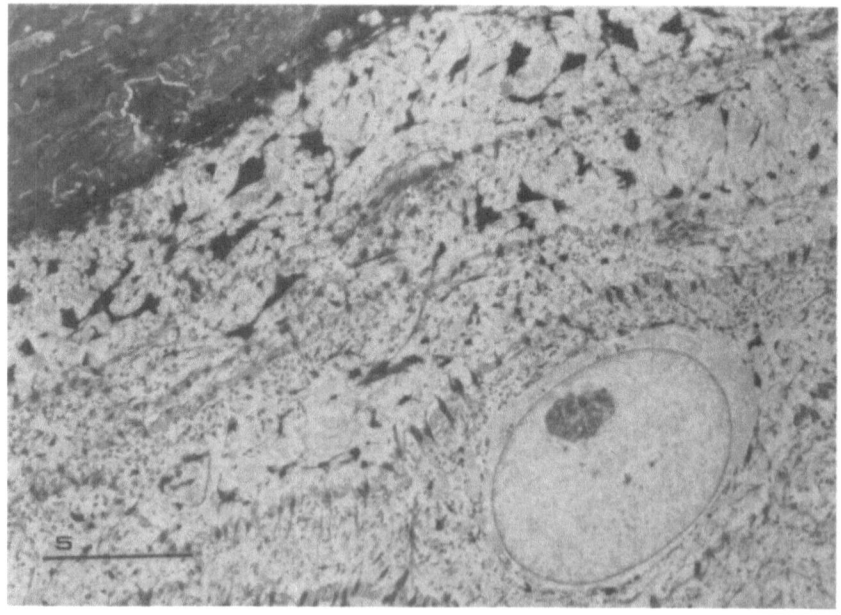

a

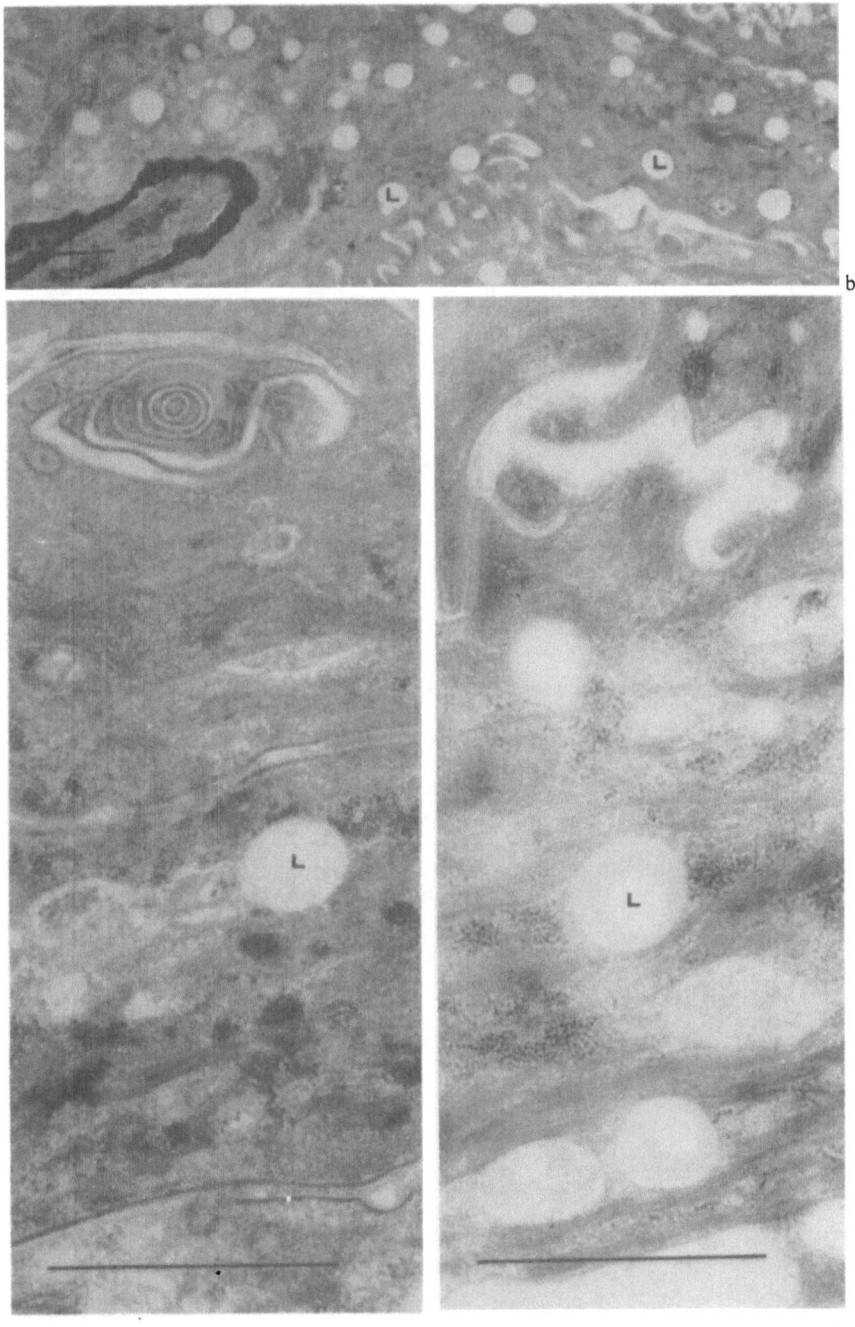

Figure 10.4   Ichthyosis congenita (lamellar ichthyosis). (a) Survey of the granular layer and lowermost horny cells; ×4 000. (b–d) Lipid droplets (L) in the horny layer; ×8 000 (b), and ×40 000 (c and d)

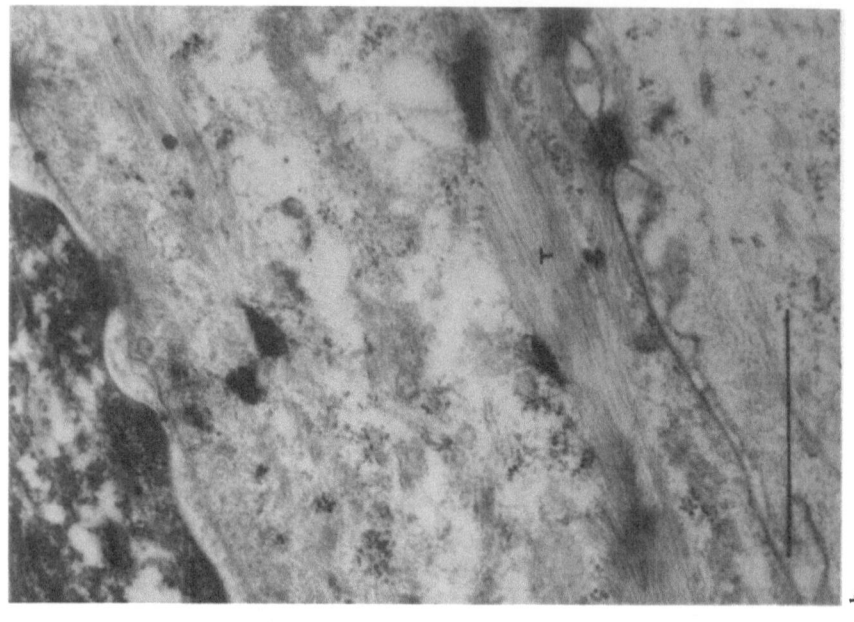

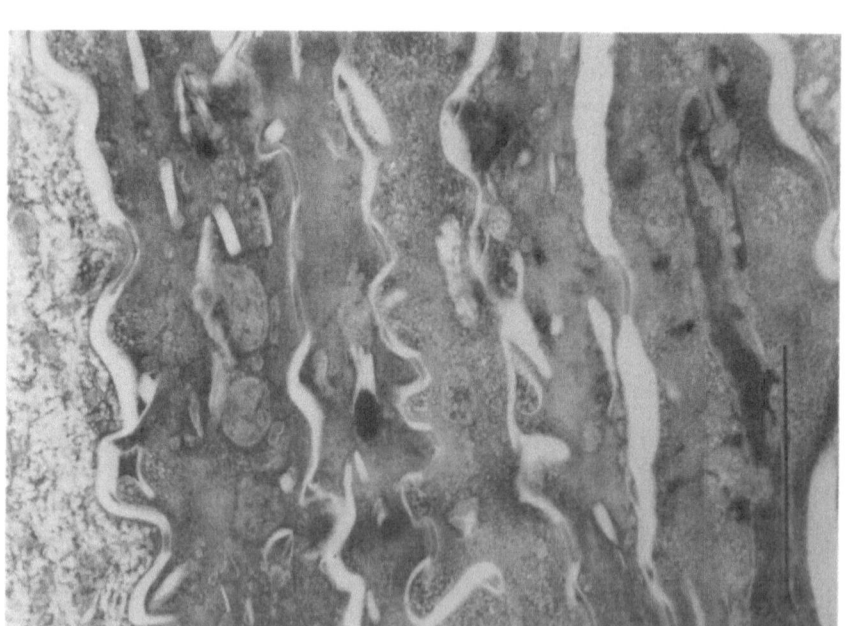

Figure 10.5 Sjögren-Larsson's syndrome. (a) Parakeratotic horny cells, no lipid inclusions present; (b) straight arrangement of tonofibrils (*T*) in a transitional cell; ×33 000

layer[13]. During keratinization desmosomes are transformed from their typical ultrastructure. The desmosomal plates that result between cornified cells are normally dissolved between the fourth to the tenth horn cell layer. The mechanism is unknown. Some lytic enzymes shown to be present in keratinosomes[17–19] may be involved in this final process of desquamation. In vulgar ichthyoses, this dissolution does not occur before the 25th to the 35th layer of horn cells[13].

ICHTHYOSIS CONGENITA GROUP

Ichthyosis congenita or lamellar ichthyosis, histologically characterized by acanthosis, hypergranulosis, ortho- and parakeratosis and varying degrees of inflammation[16] (proliferation hyperkeratosis[2]), has been shown by Frost[14,15] to exhibit increased mitotic indices and a reduced turnover time. By electron microscopy, mitoses are easily found. In the granular layer the cells are large, not normally flattened, and show merely quantitative deviations from the normal keratinization process (Figure 10.4a). Keratohyalin granules are most often small but of normal ultrastructure. A large number of well-preserved mitochondria and the occurrence of centrioles in granular cells — completely unusual in normal skin — demonstrate the immature state of these high-level keratinocytes. In parakeratotic as well as in orthokeratotic regions of the horny layer lipid droplets are a constant finding in lamellar ichthyosis (Figures 10.4b–d). They are of diagnostic value in doubtful cases[20,21].

In Sjögren-Larsson's syndrome[22], these lipid droplets were only rarely found in horny cells of two typical cases (Figure 10.5a). Another feature of Sjögren-Larsson's syndrome was stiff and very straight bundles of tonofibrils together with normal keratohyalin (Figure 10.5b). Accumulation of β-glycogene, as described by Vissian *et al.*[23] in keratinocytes of Sjögren-Larsson's syndrome, was not present in our two cases.

Ichthyosis linearis cirumflexa (Comel) will not be reported here. Frenk and Mevorah as well as Thorne and co-workers have shown that unknown substances are formed in the border of growing lesions where parakeratosis is present and keratohyalin granules are missing[24,25]. We found this process not only to be limited locally but to be restricted to short periods of abnormal differentiation (unpublished observations). In Netherton's syndrome, this type of ichthyosis is combined with trichorrhexis invaginata, the ultrastructure of which was described by Orfanos *et al.,*)[26].

HYSTRIX-LIKE ICHTHYOSES

The hystrix-like ichthyoses comprise a multitude of heterogeneous types, out of which only some few have been thoroughly investigated by electron microscopy up to now.

Bullous ichthyosiform erythroderma or epidermolytic hyperkeratosis may present with either generalized, diffuse or linear hyperkeratoses, respectively. This type of ichthyosis is characterized by an early clumping of tonofibrils that form large ring-like shells around the nuclei in the higher levels (Figure 10.6a) and result in a severely disturbed dyskeratotic horny complex[27–33,1]. Blister formation includes either acanthokeratolysis by the separation of desmosomes from one of their two neighbouring cells due to the formation of clumps of tonofibrils, followed by an enlargment of the intercellular spaces (Figure 10.6b), or cytolysis, when tonofibrillar clumps remain in contact with desmosomes (Figure 10.6c).

Ichthyosis hystrix type Curth–Macklin was first described in 1954 in two brothers[34]; the mode of transmission obviously is autosomal-dominant. By light microscopy, blown-up cells, reminiscent somewhat of epidermolytic hyperkeratosis and often binuclear, were found in the granular layer. This type is unique in the presence of unbroken concentric shells of tonofibrils, surrounding the nucleus and a region of perinuclear cytoplasm (Figure 10.7a). Binucleate cells occur throughout the epidermis in large numbers (Figure 10.7b). The tonofibrillar shells are completely different from those of epidermolytic hyperkeratosis. This type of hystrix-like ichthyosis thus represents a separate nosologic entity[35,36]. A similar, but solitary case has been described by Pinkus and Nagao[37].

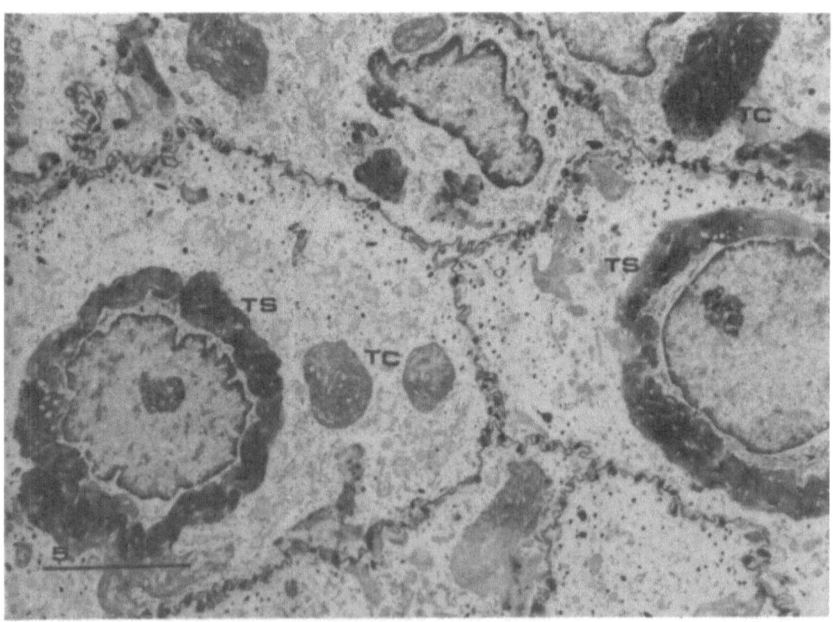

a

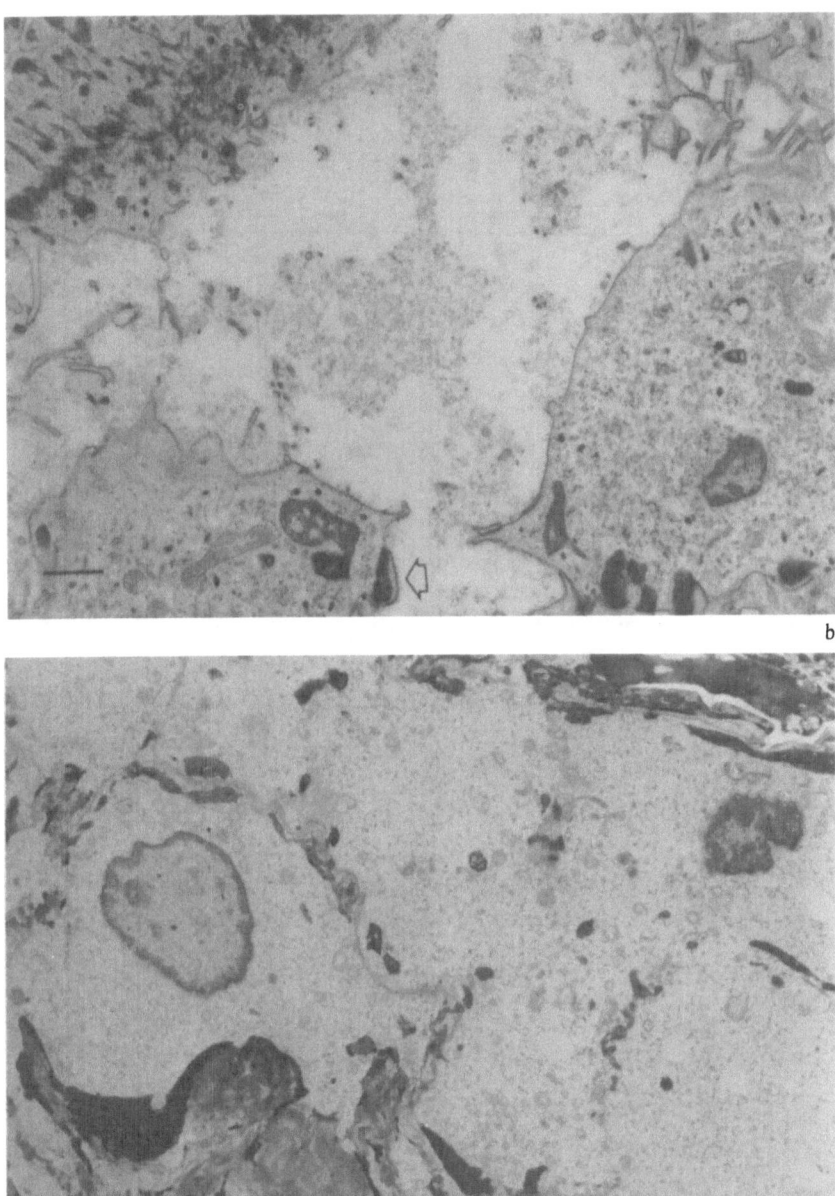

Figure 10.6 Epidermolytic hyperkeratosis. (a) Tonofibrillar clumps (*TC*) and shells (*TS*) in the uppermost prickle cell layer (compare with Figures 10.4a and 10.7b); ×4000. (b) Blister formation by acanthokeratolysis due to unilateral separation of desmosomes from one of their two neighbouring cells (open arrow) after loss of their inserting tonofilaments; ×8000. (c) Cytolytic blister formation without enlargement of intercellular spaces; ×4000

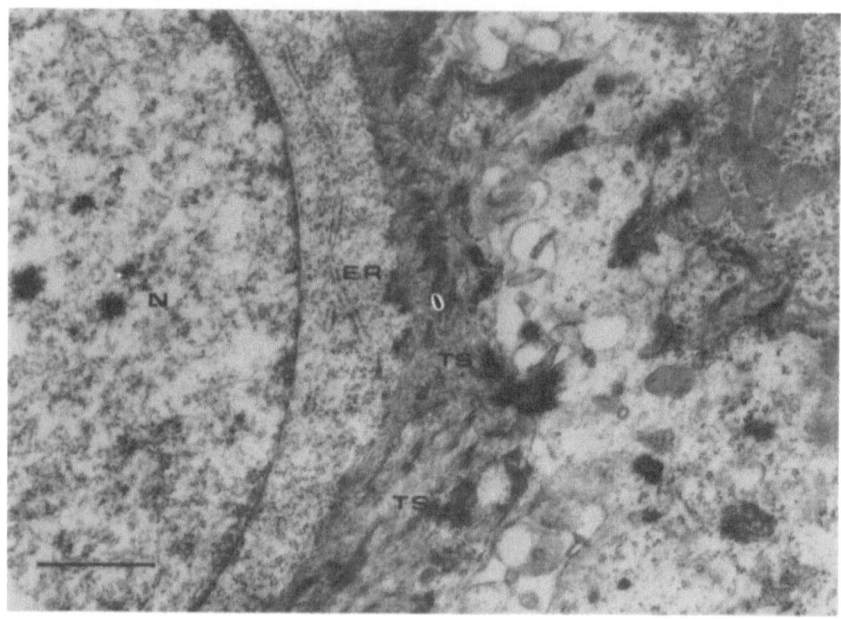

a

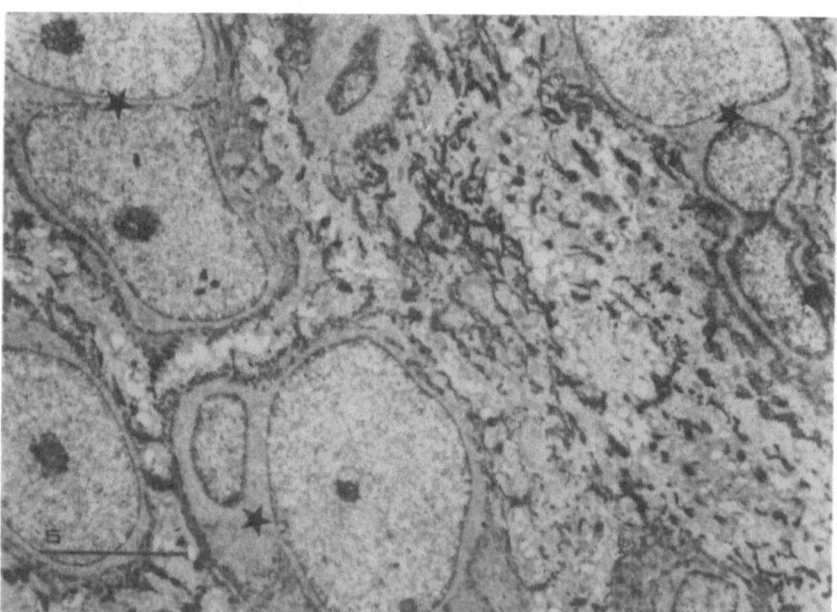

b

Figure 10.7 Ichthyosis hystrix type Curth–Macklin. (a) Unbroken concentric shell of tonofilaments (*TS*) surrounding the nucleus (*N*) and perinuclear cytoplasm with ribosomes and granular endoplasmic reticulum (*ER*); ×16 000. (b) 3 binucleate cells (★) in the prickle cell layer (compare with Figure 10.6a); ×4000

Finally, ichthyosis hystrix gravior has been reported repeatedly in the literature. It is worth remembering the famous cases of 'porcupine men' of the Lambert family[38] and the Bäfverstedt type[39,40]. A new case of ichthyosis hystrix gravior will briefly be reported. Areas of particularly severe involvement included the face, the ears, and the extremities. Skin malformation is combined in this patient with deafness of the inner ear. This patient has been demonstrated at the Dermatologic Joint Meeting at Heidelberg, October 1976[41]. He seems to us to represent a special syndrome not only from the clinical point of view but also because of his unusual ultrastructural features.

By light microscopy the epidermis shows a serrated appearance and spine-like formations. Using electron microscopy, basal cells are found to be unusually rich in organelles, Golgi bodies, and endoplasmic reticulum. Under the large spines the granular layer consists of large, blown-up cells with a central large nucleus, few keratohyalin granules, and almost no normal tono-fibrils. Instead, membrane-bound granules were found in increasing amounts in these cells. They discharge their contents to the intercellular spaces (Figure 10.8). As shown by ultrastructural enzymatic digestion experiments, they obviously contain mucous substances. In fact, histochemically a mucous metaplasia may be demonstrated in these regions. Similar mucous substances do not occur in normal human keratinizing cells. The granules resemble, however, mucous granules of frog skin. They are thought to represent a biologic compensation for the missing protective function of these highly disturbed epidermal and horny layers[42]. Because of these unique features which are not known to occur in other keratinization disorders or in normal skin, this case is regarded as representing a separate nosologic entity (type Rheydt).

CONCLUSIONS

Intrinsic ultrastructural differences exist between the various types of inherited ichthyoses that may well be used as parameters for their classification. By electron microscopy a distinction is not only possible between representatives of the main clinical groups (ichthyosis vulgaris group, congenital ichthyoses, hystrix-like ichthyoses), but also between the different types within these groups.

Structural abnormalities are demonstrable in some dominant types, in keratohyalin (defective in autosomal dominant ichthyosis vulgaris), and tono-filaments (impaired or disturbed in their arrangement in hystrix-like ichthyoses: clump formation in bullous ichthyosiform erythroderma or epidermolytic hyperkeratosis; shell formation associated with high numbers of binucleate cells in ichthyosis hystrix type Curth–Macklin; impairment in ichthyosis hystrix gravior type Rheydt). Keratohyalin and tonofilaments are both structural proteins of keratinizing tissues.

In most recessive types merely quantitative deviations from the normal keratinization process have been found (X-linked recessive ichthyosis, lamellar

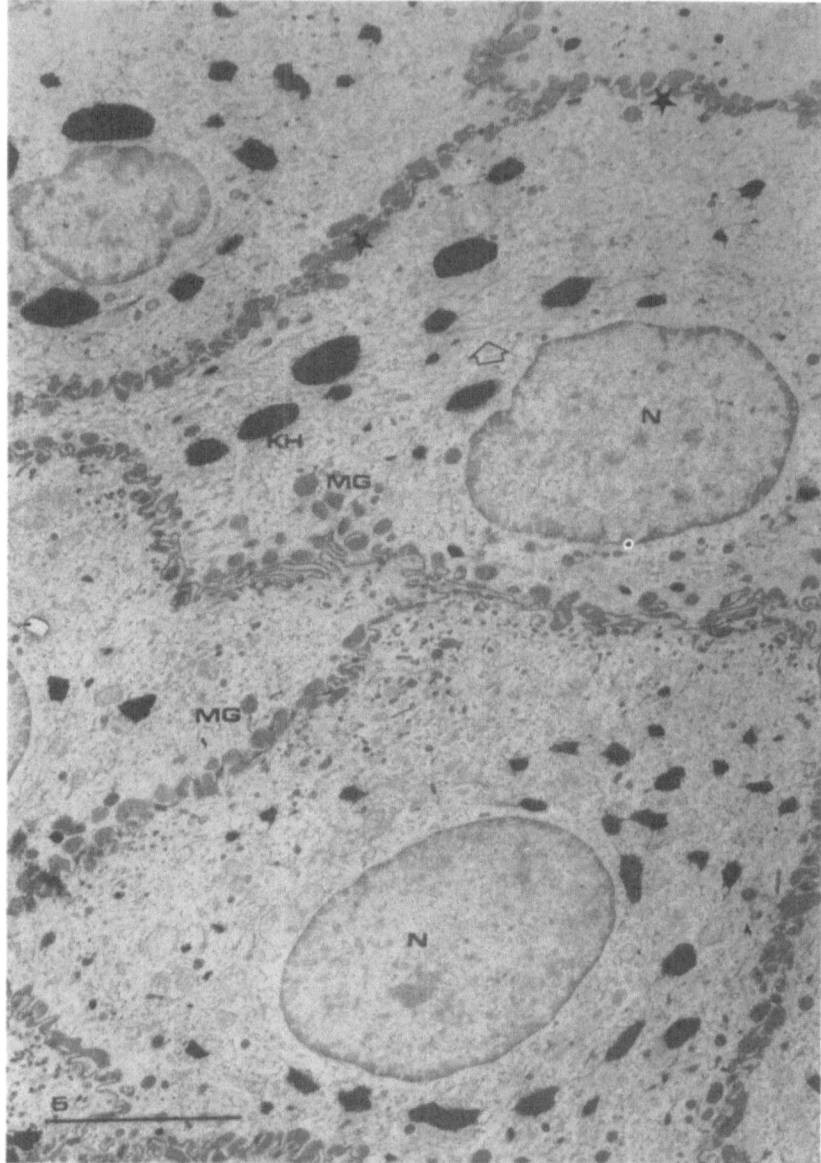

Figure 10.8 Ichthyosis hystrix gravior with deafness (Type Rheydt). Blown-up cells of the granular layer with largely reduced amounts of tonofilaments (open arrow), normal or slightly rounded keratohyalin (*KH*) granules, and production of membrane-bound mucous granules (*MG*) that discharge their contents to the intercellular spaces (★); *N*–nuclei; ×5500

ichthyosis, Sjögren-Larsson's syndrome, Refsum's syndrome). In Refsum's syndrome, lipid droplets representing storage of phytanic acid due to a defective α-oxidation are demonstrable in keratinocytes and melanocytes of ichthyotic skin, whereas in lamellar ichthyosis lipid vacuoles are regularly present in horny cells.

Thus, clinically very similar types of inherited ichthyoses may be separated by their distinctive morphologic differences[1]. It may be expected that future ultrastructural studies will reveal the existence of further heterogeneities in the inherited ichthyoses. Moreover, electron microscopy has become a valuable tool in their exact diagnosis and is of great importance for our understanding of the kind of disturbances that lead to these types of 'inborn errors of keratinization'.

References

1. Anton-Lamprecht, I. and Schnyder, U. W. (1974). Ultrastructure of inborn errors of keratinization. VI. Inherited ichthyoses — a model system for heterogeneities in keratinization disturbances. *Arch. Dermatol. Forsch.*, **250**, 207
2. Schnyder, U. W. (1970). Inherited ichthyoses. *Arch. Dermatol.*, **102**, 240
3. Schnyder, U. W. (1974). Inherited disorders of the skin and skin disorders due to a hereditary predisposition. *J. Dermatol.*, **1**, 65
4. Elias, P. M. and Friend, D. S. (1975). The permeability barrier in mammalian epidermis. *J. Cell Biol.*, **65**, 180
5. Wells, R. S. and Kerr, C. B. (1966). The histology of ichthyosis. *J. Invest. Dermatol.*, **46**, 530
6. Kuokkanen, K. (1969). Ichthyosis vulgaris. A clinical and histopathological study of patients and their close relatives in the autosomal dominant and sex-linked forms of the disease. *Acta Dermatol.-Venereol. (Stockholm)*, **49** (Suppl. 62), 1
7. Woźniak, C. and Omulecki, A. (1970). Unterscheidungsmerkmale der x-chromosomalen rezessiven und der autosomalen dominanten Ichthyosis vulgaris. *Dermatol. Mschr.*, **156**, 503
8. Feinstein, A., Ackerman, A. B. and Ziprkowski, L. (1970). Histology of autosomal dominant ichthyosis vulgaris and x-linked ichthyosis. *Arch. Dermatol.*, **101**, 524
9. Hofbauer, M. and Schnyder, U. W. (1974). Zur Differentialdiagnose von autosomal-dominanter Ichthyosis vulgaris und X-chromosomaler Ichthyose. *Hautarzt*, **25**, 319
10. Anton-Lamprecht, I. (1974). Zur Ultrastruktur hereditärer Verhornungsstörungen. IV. X-chromosomal-rezessive Ichthyosis. *Arch. Dermatol. Forsch.*, **248**, 361
11. Anton-Lamprecht, I. (1973). Zur Ultrastruktur hereditärer Verhornungsstörungen. III. Autosomal-dominante Ichthyosis vulgaris. *Arch. Dermatol. Forsch.*, **248**, 149
12. Anton-Lamprecht, I. and Hofbauer, M. (1972). Ultrastructural distinction of autosomal dominant ichthyosis vulgaris and X-linked recessive ichthyosis. *Humangenetik*, **15**, 261
13. Anton-Lamprecht, I. and Kahlke, W. (1974). Zur Ultrastruktur hereditärer Verhornungsstörungen. V. Ichthyosis beim Refsum-Syndrom (Heredopathia atactica polyneuritiformis). *Arch. Dermatol. Forsch.*, **250**, 185
14. Frost, P. and Weinstein, G. D. (1971). Ichthyosiform dermatoses. In T. B. Fitzpatrick (ed.). *Dermatology in General medicine*, pp. 249–265 (New York: McGraw-Hill Inc.)
15. Frost, P. (1973). Ichthyosiform dermatoses. *J. Invest. Dermatol.*, **60**, 541
16. Schnyder, U. W. and Konrad, B. (1967). Zur Histogenetik der Ichthyosen. *Hautarzt*, **18**, 445

17. Wolff, K. and Holubar, K. (1967). Odland-Körper (Membrane coating granules, Keratinosomen) als epidermale Lysosomen. Ein elektronenmikroskopisch-cytochemischer Beitrag zum Verhornungsprozess der Haut. *Arch. Klin. Exp. Dermatol.*, **231**, 1

18. Weinstock, M. and Wilgram, G. F. (1970). Fine-structural observations on the formation and enzymatic activity of keratinosomes in mouse tongue filiform papillae. *J. Ultrastruct. Res.*, **30**, 262

19. Takaki, Y. (1971). An electron microscopic study of membrane coating granules in normal skin and abnormal keratinization with reference to acid phosphatase activity. *Jap. J. Dermatol., B.*, **81**, 131

20. Anton-Lamprecht, I. (1972). Zur Ultrastruktur hereditärer Verhornungsstörungen. I. Ichthyosis congenita. *Arch. Dermatol. Forsch.*, **243**, 88

21. Vandersteen, P. R. and Muller, S. A. (1972). Lamellar ichthyosis. An enzyme histochemical, light, and electron microscopic study. *Arch. Dermatol.*, **106**, 694

22. Theile, U. (1974). Sjögren-Larsson Syndrome. Oligophrenia — Ichthyosis — Di/Tetraplegia. *Humangenetik*, **22**, 91

23. Vissian, L., Raibaudi, R. and Vaillaud, J. C. (1971). Syndrome de Sjögren-Larsson chez un nourrisson. *Bull. Soc. Fr. Dermatol. Syphiligr.*, **78**, 500

24. Frenk, E. and Mevorah, B. (1972). Ichthyosis linearis circumflexa Comèl with trichorrhexis invaginata (Netherton's syndrome). An ultrastructural study of skin changes. *Arch. Dermatol. Forsch.*, **245**, 42

25. Thorne, E. G., Zelickson, A. S., Mottaz, J. H., Katz, H. I. and Deaton, B. H. (1975). Netherton's syndrome. An electron microscopic study. *Arch. Dermatol. Res.*, **253**, 177

26. Orfanos, C. E., Mahrle, G. and Šalomon, T. (1971). Netherton Syndrom. Ichthyosiforme Hautveränderungen und Trichorrhexis invaginata. Nachweis eines krankhaft veränderten Cortexkeratins im Haar. *Hautarzt*, **22**, 397

27. Weibel, E. R. and Schnyder, U. W. (1966). Zur Ultrastruktur und Histochemie der granulösen Degeneration bei bullöser Erythrodermie congénitale ichthyosiforme. *Arch. Klin. Exp. Dermatol.*, **225**, 286

28. Wilgram, G. F. and Caulfield, J. B. (1966). An electron microscopic study of epidermolytic hyperkeratosis. With a special note on the keratinosome as the 'fourth' structural factor in the formation of the horny layer. *Arch. Dermatol.*, **94**, 127

29. Wilgram, G. F. and Weinstock, A. (1966). Advances in genetic dermatology. Dyskeratosis, acantholysis, and hyperkeratosis. With a special note on the specific role of desmosomes and keratinosomes in the formation of the horny layer. *Arch. Dermatol.*, **94**, 456

30. Ishibashi, Y. and Klingmüller, G. (1968). Erythrodermia ichthyosiformis congenita bullosa Brocq. Über die sogenannte granulöse Degeneration. I–V. *Arch. Klin. Exp. Dermatol.*, **231**, 424; **232**, 205; **233**, 11; **233**, 107; **233**, 124

31. Hirone, T. (1969). Electron microscopic studies of ichthyosis and congenital ichthyosiform erythroderma. *J. Electr. Microsc.*, **18**, 63

32. Orfanos, C. E. (1972). *Feinstrukturelle Morphologie und Histopathologie der verhornenden Epidermis.* (Stuttgart: Thieme)

33. Blanchet-Bardon, C., Anton-Lamprecht, I. and Schnyder, U. W. (1977). Erythrodermie congénitale ichthyosiforme bulleuse — contrôle ultrastructural du traitement par un dérivé éthylique de l'acide rétinoique. *Ann. Dermatol. Syph.* (Paris) (In press)

34. Curth, H. O. and Macklin, M. T. (1954). The genetic basis of various types of ichthyosis in a family group. *Am. J. Hum. Genet.*, **6**, 371

35. Ollendorff-Curth, H., Allen, F. H., Schnyder, U. W. and Anton-Lamprecht, I. (1972). Follow-up of a family group suffering from ichthyosis hystrix type Curth–Macklin. *Humangenetik*, **17**, 37

36. Anton-Lamprecht, I., Curth, H. O. and Schnyder, U. W. (1973). Zur Ultrastruktur hereditärer Verhornungsstörungen. II. Ichthyosis hystrix Typ Curth–Macklin. *Arch. Dermatol. Forsch.*, **246**, 77

37. Pinkus, H. and Nagao, S. (1970). A case of biphasic ichthyosiform dermatosis: light and electron microscopic study. *Arch. Klin. Exp. Dermatol.*, **237,** 737
38. Penrose, C. S. and Stern, C. (1958). Reconsideration of the Lambert pedigree (ichthyosis hystrix gravior). *Ann. Hum. Genet.*, **22,** 258
39. Bäfverstedt, B. (1941). Fall von genereller, naevusartiger Hyperkeratose, Imbecillität, Epilepsie, *Acta Dermatol.-Venereol. (Stockh.*), **22,** 207
40. Lodin, A. and Gentele, H. (1958). Maleformatio ectodermalis generalisata: Hyperkeratosis follicularis monstruosa: Imbecillitas; Epilepsia. In *One Hundred Clinical Cases*, presented at the 11th Intern. Congr. of Dermatol., Stockholm, 1957, pp. 108–109 (Stockholm: Acta Dermato-Venereologica cop.)
41. Schnyder, U. W., Gloor, M., Anton-Lamprecht, I., Bersch, A., Böhm, W., Schöpf, E., Schröter, R. and Tilgen, W. (1977). Krankendemonstration, Gemeinschaftstagung der Südwestdeutschen Dermatologen-Vereinigung und der Vereinigung Rheinisch-Westfälischer Dermatologen, Heidelberg 1976. *Z. Hautkr.*, **52,** 763
42. Anton-Lamprecht, I. (1976). Biologic compensation for missing protective function of the skin due to congenital lack of tonofibrils. *J. Invest. Dermatol.*, **66,** 259

11
Preliminary Freeze-Fracture Observations in Ichthyosis Vulgaris

R. CAPUTO, M. INNOCENTI, G. GASPARINI and D. PELUCHETTI

ABSTRACT

Freeze-fracture study of two cases of ichthyosis vulgaris has revealed:

— the absence or a small number of gap junctions
— an increase in tight junctions in the spinous layer
— an increase in the number of keratinosomes showing a normal appearance

The absence or small number of gap junctions can be attributed to a vitamin A deficiency. A higher number of tight junctions can be interpreted as an attempt to make up for the decrease in the barrier function of the most superficial layers, which is probably the consequence of a modification of the lipid component of keratinosomes.

Ichthyosis vulgaris is a retention hyperkeratosis[1], ultrastructurally characterized[2,3] by the absence of the granular layer or by keratohyalin granules which are abnormal, being small and spongy. However, the hyperkeratotic horny layer reveals a normal pattern. In spite of the fact that the number of keratinosomes is unchanged[3] and that the stacking pattern of the horny cells is normal[4], a decrease of the barrier function has also been demonstrated in this disease[5]. We have employed the freeze-fracture technique for the purpose of gathering new information on the inner structure of cell membranes and cell junctions, as well as on the barrier function.

MATERIALS AND METHODS

Biopsy fragments of two cases of ichthyosis vulgaris were fixed with 3% glutaraldehyde in phosphate buffer 0.12 M, pH 7.3, for 2–3 hours, and then infiltrated in 10%–20%–30% glycerol buffered with phosphate 0.12 M, pH 7.3. The samples were frozen by immersion in Freon 22, cooled to −150 °C in liquid nitrogen and then freeze-fractured according to the method of Moor *et al.*[6] in a Balzers freeze-etching device. The fracturing temperature was −115 °C. Platinum carbon replicas were washed first in Na-hypochlorite to remove the organic material, and then in distilled water, and recovered on 200-mesh grids. The replicas were examined with Philips EM 200 and EM 300 electron microscopes.

RESULTS

The examination of the replicas from the two cases of ichthyosis vulgaris under study has led to the following observations: The number of membrane associated particles and the appearance of the desmosomes are unchanged as compared to normal epidermis; Gap junctions are absent in one case, while they are small and very rare in the other case; In both cases, many tight junctions can be found in the spinous layer (Figure 11.1), which are seldom observed in normal epidermis; Keratinosomes are quite numerous in the most

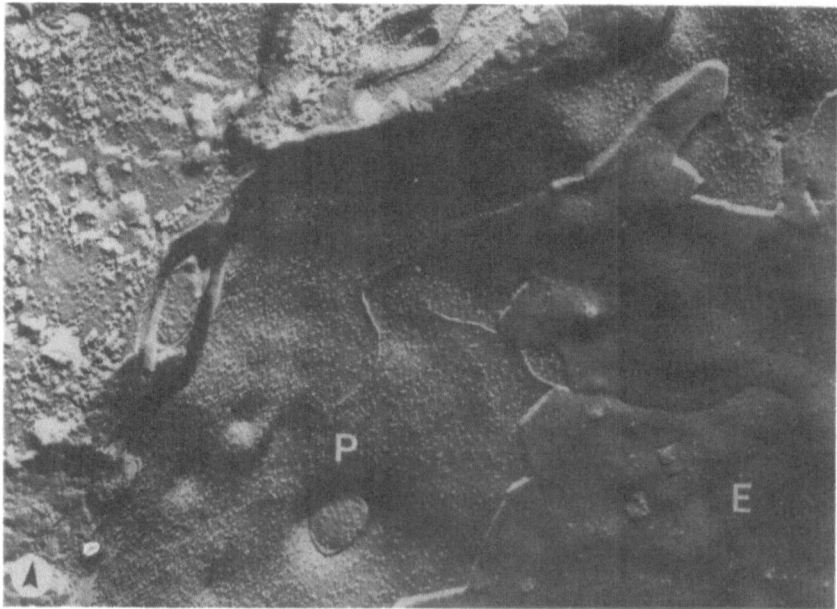

Figure 11.1 Typical tight junction (ridges on the *P* face and grooves on the *E* face) between two cells of the spinous layer (×28 000)

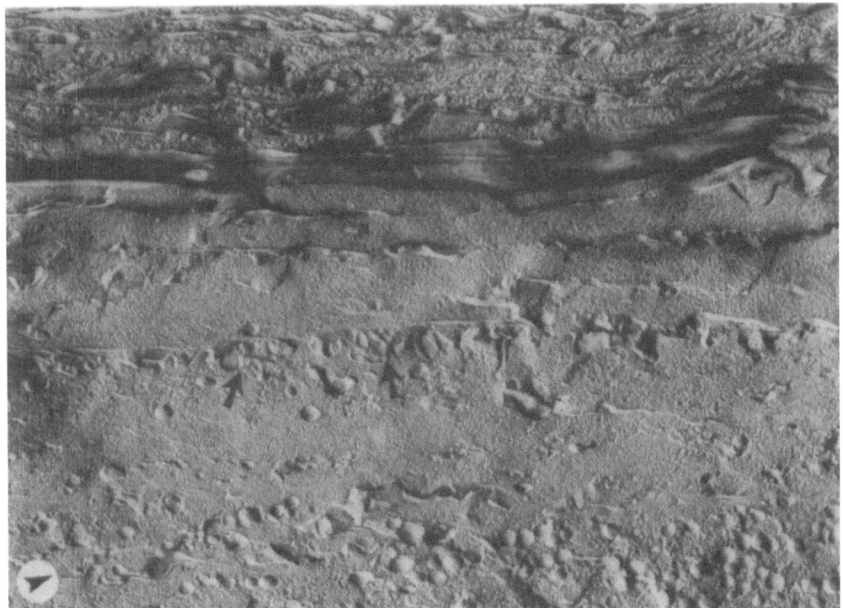

Figure 11.2 Transition area between the spinous and horny layers. Keratinosomes are numerous also in intercellular spaces (arrows) (×16 100)

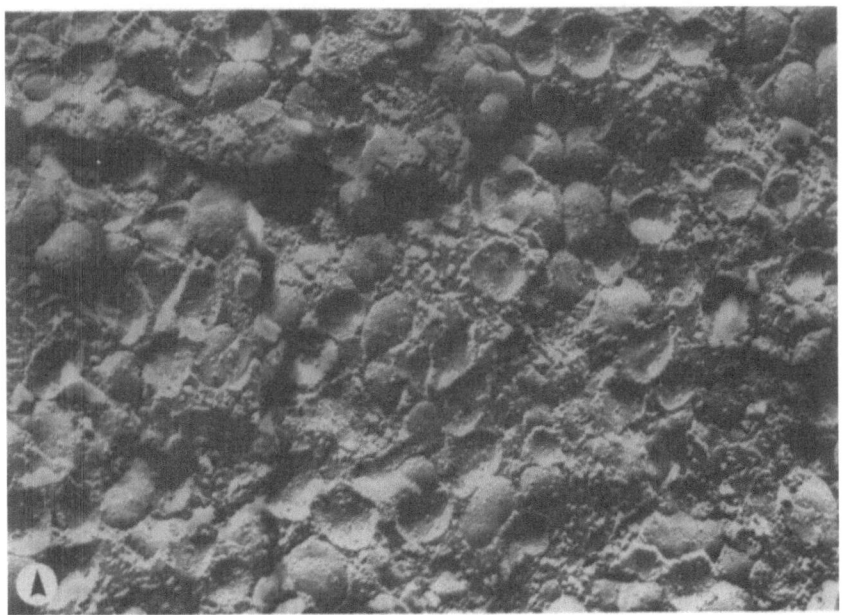

Figure 11.3 High magnification of a group of keratinosomes in the spinous layer. Many *P* (concave) and *E* (convex) faces of the limiting membrane of the granule can be seen (×50 400)

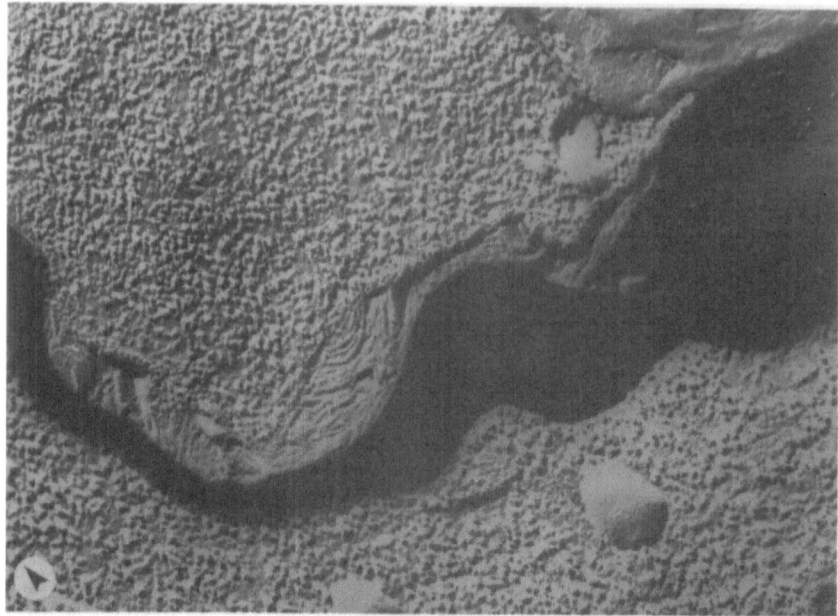

Figure 11.4 Cells of the horny layer. The intercellular space is filled by the content of keratinosomes, exhibiting a lamellar organization (×63 200)

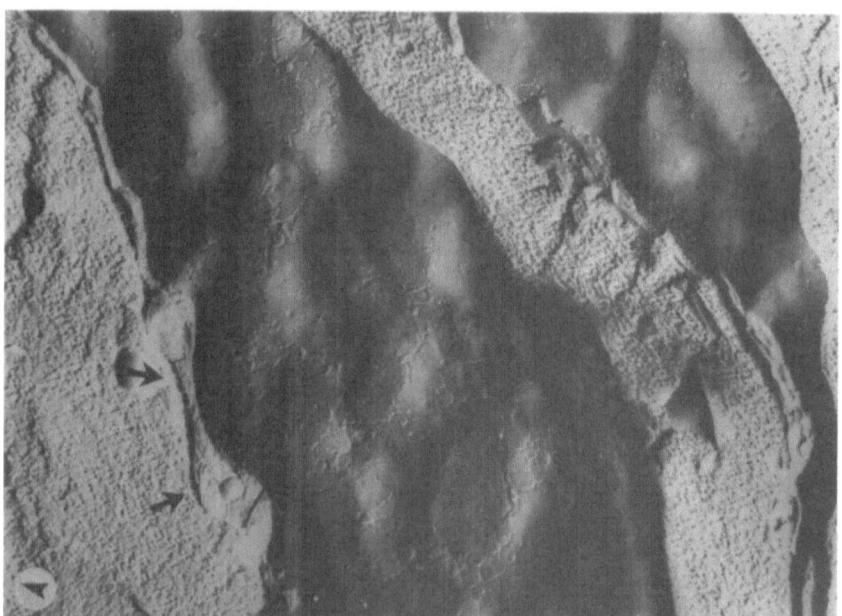

Figure 11.5 First cells of the horny layer. A ridges pattern in connection with the desmosomes can be observed on the *E* face. The arrows indicate the lamellar material poured by keratinosomes into intercellular spaces (×32 500)

superficial layers of the spinous layer (Figure 11.2). They were found to be three times as many as those present in normal epidermis. The keratinosomes look concave when the P face is exposed, since the granule has been, so to speak, enucleated; they look convex when the E face is exposed, since the fracture plane runs as if it were peeling the granule (Figure 11.3). These organelles are easily observable in intercellular spaces, also in the horny layer (Figure 11.4). The high number of these organelles in intercellular spaces is probably responsible for the many fracture jumps observed between the membranes of adjacent cells, in the most superficial layers of the horny layer. In the first cells of the horny layer, the typical membrane specializations observed in normal epidermis can be found[7], but they are more disorganized (Figure 11.5).

DISCUSSION

In the replicas, the unmodified number of membrane associated particles is no surprise, since this disease shows a normal mitotic index[1]. The usual arrangement of membrane associated particles in correspondence with the desmosomes substantiates thin section observations. On the contrary, the absence or the low number of gap junctions found is an interesting fact. This phenomenon can possibly be ascribed to a vitamin A deficiency since, as is well known, this substance stimulates the synthesis of glycoproteins and RNA[8], binds to plasma proteins[9] and has been experimentally shown to induce the formation of gap junctions[10].

In thin section, investigations show that the number of keratinosomes appears to be either unmodified[3] or decreased[11]; in the replicas, their number was found to be three times as high as the normal one. This counting is probably more accurate than those which are carried out on thin sections, since with the freeze-fracture technique the influence of the 'thickness' factor is eliminated.

The limiting membrane of keratinosomes retains its normal appearance. Keratinosomes are clearly evident in intercellular spaces and exhibits a lamellar organization. The freeze-fracture technique, which is particularly useful in the study of cell membranes, has provided no new information on the structure of keratohyalin.

In spite of the fact that the morphological equivalents of the barrier function (keratinosomes[12] and the typical membrane specializations of the first cells of the horny layer[7]) are present in good number, physiological investigations have shown a modification of this function in ichthyosis[1]. It can therefore be hypothesized that the decrease in the barrier function is due to a qualitative (not quantitative) modification of the lipid component of keratinosomes, which is discharged into intercellular spaces and which, in normal epidermis, represents an ideal impermeable barrier[12]. The increase in the number of tight junctions between the cells of the spinous layer might be interpreted as an attempt to make up for this barrier deficit of the most superficial layers.

Acknowledgements

The authors are greatly indebted to P. Tinelli and F. Crippa for technical help.

References

1. Frost, P., Weinstein, G. D. and Van Scott, E. J. (1966). The ichthyosiform dermatoses. II. Autoradiographic studies of epidermal proliferation. *J. Invest. Dermatol.*, **47**, 561
2. Anton-Lamprecht, I. (1973). Zur Ultrastruktur hereditärer Verhornungsstörungen. III. Autosomal-dominante Ichthyosis vulgaris. *Arch. Dermatol. Forsch.*, **248**, 149
3. Anton-Lamprecht, I. and Schnyder, V. W. (1974). Ultrastructure of inborn errors of keratinization. IV. Inherited ichthyoses. A model system for heterogeneities in keratinization disturbances. *Arch. Dermatol. Forsch.*, **250**, 207
4. Menton, D. N. and Eisen, A. Z. (1971). Structural organization of the stratum corneum in certain scaling disorders of the skin. *J. Invest. Dermatol.*, **57**, 295
5. Frost, P., Weinstein, G. D., Bothwell, J. W. and Wildnauer, R. (1968). Ichthyosiform dermatoses. III. Studies of transepidermal water loss. *Arch. Dermatol.*, **98**, 230
6. Moor, H., Muhlethaler, K., Waldner, H. and Frey-Wysshug, A. (1961). A new freezing ultramicrotome. *J. Biophys. Biochem. Cytol.*, **10**, 1
7. Caputo, R. and Peluchetti, D. (1975). The junctions of normal human epidermis. A freeze-fracture study. Presented at the Joint Meeting of the Society for Investigative Dermatology and of the European Society of Dermatological Research, Amsterdam, June 9–13, 1975
8. De Luca, L. and Yuspa, S. H. (1974). Altered glycoprotein synthesis in mouse epidermal cells treated with retinyl acetate in vitro. *Exp. Cell Res.*, **86**, 106
9. Kanal, M., Raz, A. and Goodman, W. S. (1968). Retinol-binding protein: the transport protein for vitamin A in human plasma. *J. Clin. Invest.*, **47**, 2025
10. Elias, P. and Friend, D. S. (1976). Vitamin A-induced mucous metaplasia. *J. Cell Biol.*, **68**, 173
11. Takaky, Y. (1971). An electron microscopic study of membrane coating granules in normal skin and abnormal keratinization with reference to acid phosphatase activity. *Jap. J. Dermatol.*, **81**, 372
12. Lavker, R. (1976). Membrane coating granules: the fate of the discharged lamellae. *J. Ultrastruct. Res.*, **55**, 79

12
Morphological and Quantitative Assessment of Physical Changes in the Horny Layer in Ichthyosis

S. NICHOLLS, C. S. KING and R. MARKS

ABSTRACT

Techniques are described which assess morphological and physical changes in ichthyotic stratum corneum. Replicas of the skin surface were viewed by scanning electron microscopy and an abnormality in desquamation was seen which suggested a greater adherence than usual between ichthyotic squames. An instrument was employed to measure the force required to remove partial thickness horny layer *in vivo* (cohesography). There was greater intracorneal cohesion in patients with severe ichthyosis than in normals. Skin surface biopsies taken from these patients revealed abnormal tracings when examined and measured in a surfometer which also suggested a greater than usual intracorneal cohesion. An X-ray probe microanalyser within a scanning electron microscope was used to investigate the distribution of elements in ichthyotic and normal stratum corneum and preliminary results suggested an abnormal distribution of sulphur and potassium in the former.

INTRODUCTION

The major types of ichthyotic disorders may reflect a disorder of desquamation or keratinization. There is a loss of plasticity of the horny layer and this results in fissuring of the skin surface. So far no striking abnormalities have been detected in epidermal growth or biochemical activity and it seems likely that the predominant change is in the stratum corneum and/or the granular cell layers alone. We now wish to report observations made on the surface morphology and physical properties of the ichthyotic stratum cornuem (S.C.).

MATERIALS AND METHODS

Surface morphology — skin surface replica production

Silfo rubber impression material (J. E. S. Davies Ltd., London) was used to obtain 'negative' impressions of the skin surface of normal and ichthyotic subjects. Sarkany and Caron (1965)[1] described how this material may be employed in the investigation of surface microtopography.

In our study 2 ml of Silfo was mixed with 2 drops of the catalyst and applied to the skin surface. It was peeled off after 1–2 minutes when dry and subsequently covered with a thin smear of 'DPX' (R. A. Lamb, London) — a styrene based slide mounting medium, and placed in a desiccator for 6 hours. The surface replicas were then removed from the rubber base. These were then 'sputter' coated with gold in a Polaron, E 5000 coater and viewed in a Cambridge scanning electron microscope (SEM) stereoscan, Mark II. Replicas of S.C. from patients with dominant ichthyosis, a patient with Refsum's syndrome and normal controls were studied.

Physical properties

Cohesography

Desquamation results from the controlled loss of cohesion between squames and we have attempted to quantitate this intracorneal cohesion using an apparatus which measures stratum corneum breaking strength *in vivo*[2]. The method, termed 'cohesography', involves the sticking of a removable circular metal head (50 mm² area) to the skin surface with a cyanoacrylate adhesive (Permabond–Staident Ltd., Staines, Middlesex). A manually driven piston pulls the head vertically from the skin, removing partial thickness horn from the area of contact. The force (in g) is measured by a transducer and the charge amplified and measured on a chart recorder.

Surfometry

Skin surface biopsies (SSBs) were taken from the arms (flexor and extensor aspects) of 5 patients with severe dominant ichthyosis using the technique of Marks and Dawber[3]. The SSB reveals the ruptured internal surface of the horny layer which partially reflects the internal cohesive forces in the S.C.[2].

The contours of this surface were traced by a fine stylus of an apparatus called a surfometer[4]. The areas beneath 10 cm lengths of surfometer tracings were measured with a planimeter.

Energy dispersive analysis of X-rays

An X-ray probe microanalyser attached to a Cambridge scanning electron microscope was used to examine the element distribution in the S.C. of SSBs. The analysis is from the surface and the top 1 μm of the specimen. The underlying adhesive does not affect the spectra obtained[5]. Each element has a characteristic X-ray energy which can be detected and measured. We have made preliminary observations on the element distribution spectra in normal S.C. and from a patient with dominant ichthyosis.

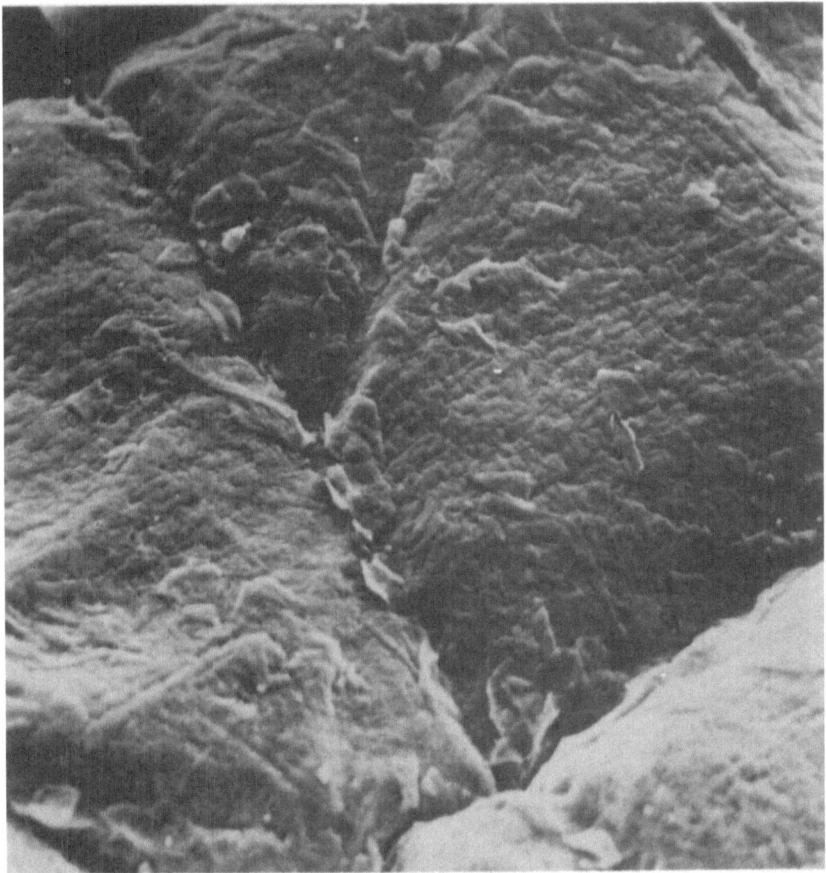

Figure 12.1 Scanning electron micrograph (SEM) of a skin surface replica taken from a normal forearm (×212)

RESULTS

Scanning electron micrographs of skin surface replicas

Replicas of normal S.C. showed individual corneocytes and small groups of partially detached corneocytes which seemed about to desquamate (Figure 12.1). Replicas from the skin of patients with dominant ichthyosis showed corneocytes which were closely adherent to the surface of the replica and large clumps of corneocytes detaching *en masse* (Figure 12.2). In addition cracking and fissuring was observed in most of the ichthyotic specimens. This was particularly noticeable on the replica taken from the patient with Refsum's syndrome (Figure 12.3).

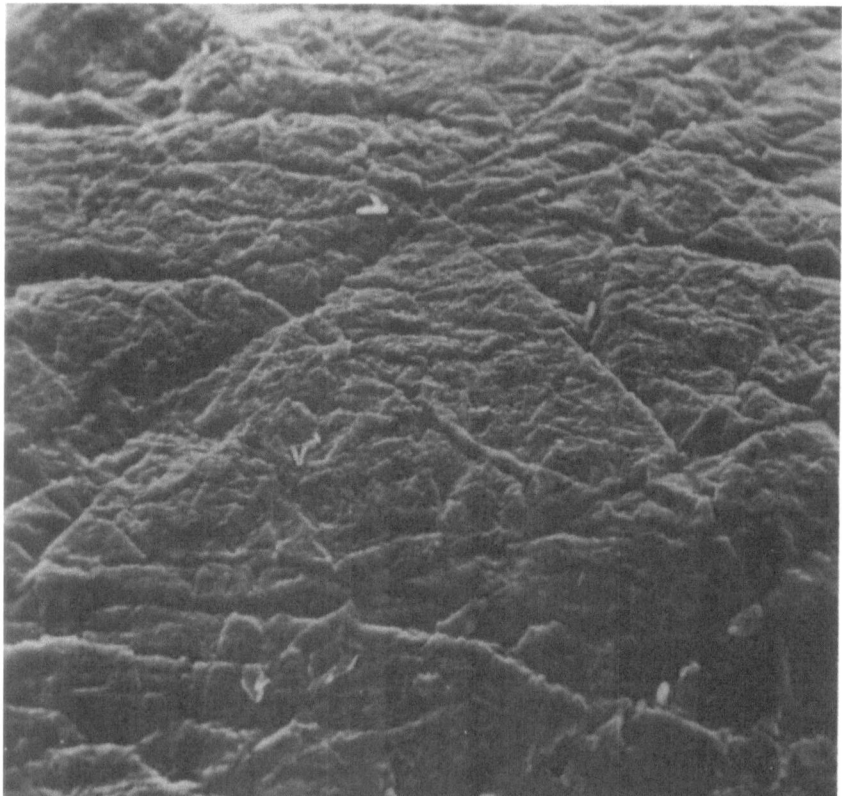

Figure 12.2 SEM of a skin surface replica from the upper arm of a patient with severe dominant ichthyosis ($\times 209$)

Cohesography

Table 12.1 shows the force required to remove partial thickness horn from normals and patients with severe dominant ichthyosis. The difference in the values is significant ($P < 0.01$).

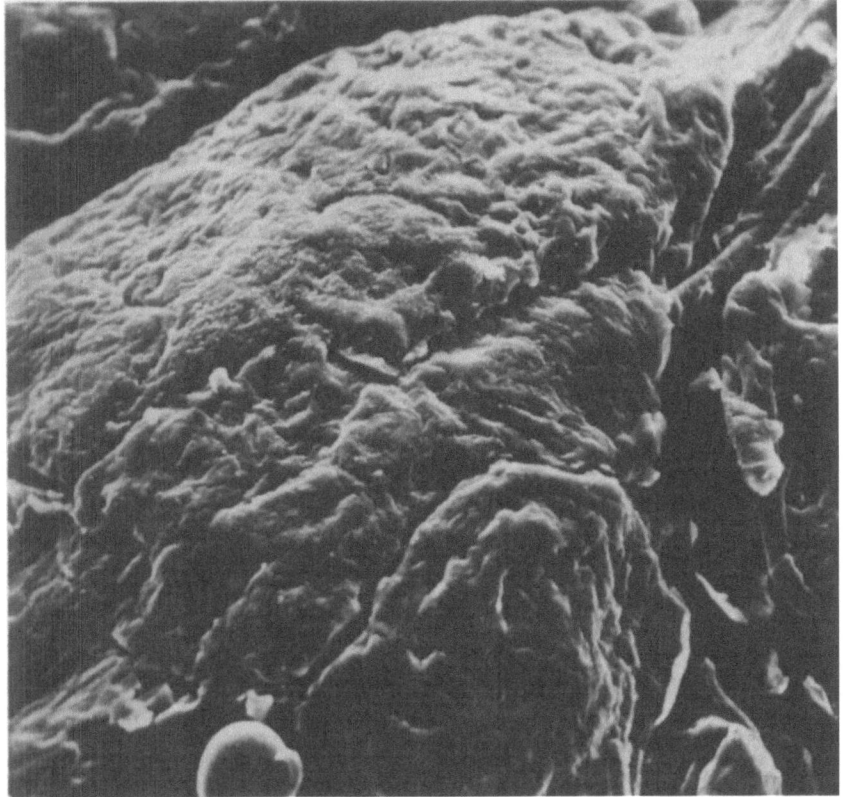

Figure 12.3 SEM of a skin surface replica from the forearm of a patient with Refsum's syndrome (×182)

Table 12.1 Cohesography force required to remove partial thickness stratum corneum from the forearm of normal subjects and patients with dominant ichthyosis

	Mean cohesive force ± standard deviation (g)
Normals ($n = 10$)	95.2 ± 17.3
Dominant ichthyosis ($n = 5$)	153.1 ± 43.8*

* Significantly different from normal ($P < 0.01$).

Surfometry

The differences between the appearances of the surfometry tracings from the SSBs derived from normal individuals and those from patients with severe dominant ichthyosis were marked. Examples are given in Figure 12.4. Mean areas of the surfometry tracings from the 5 ichthyotic specimens were

SURFOMETRY

NORMAL TRACE

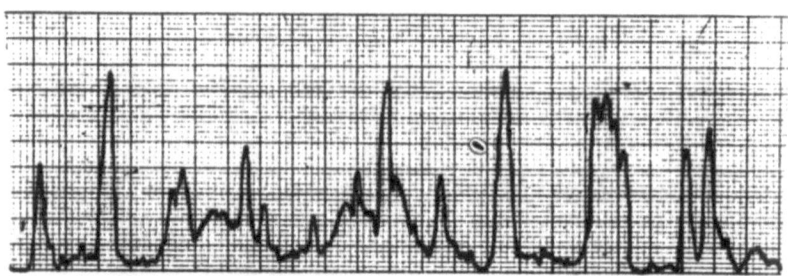

ICHTHYOSIS VULGARIS

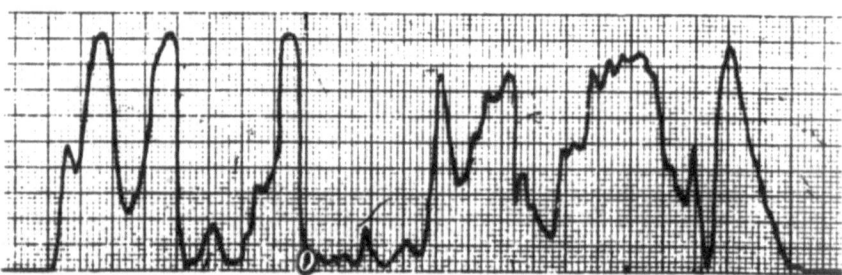

Figure 12.4 Comparison of surfometry tracings from skin surface biopsies (SSB) of a normal individual and a patient with severe dominant ichthyosis

compared to the areas of ten normal subjects (Table 12.2). The difference in the values obtained is significant ($P < 0.01$).

Table 12.2 Surfometry: Comparison of surfometric areas in SSB's from normal subjects and patients with ichthyosis

	Mean surfometric area in 10 cm trace ± standard deviation
Normals ($n = 10$)	8.9 ± 0.97
Dominant ichthyosis ($n = 5$)	$13.3 \pm 4.1^*$

* Significantly different for normal ($P < 0.01$).

Energy dispersive analysis

Figure 12.5 illustrates the element spectrum derived from the energy dispersive analysis of an SSB from a normal subject. Large amounts of chlorine, potassium and small amounts of sulphur are indicated. The smaller peaks on the left

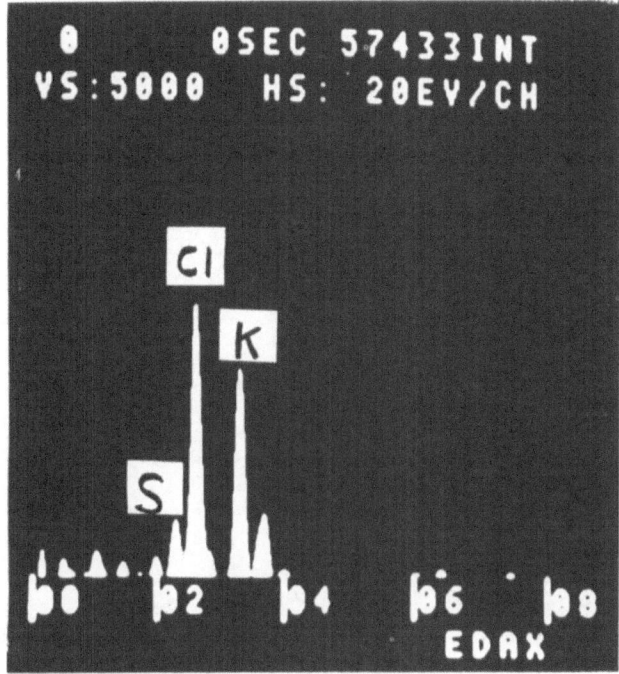

Figure 12.5 An element spectrum derived from energy dispersive analysis of SSB from a normal subject (Cl = chlorine, K = potassium, S = sulphur)

of the spectrum represent elements such as sodium and magnesium. Figure 12.6 shows the element spectrum derived from an SSB taken from a patient with dominant ichthyosis. The sulphur levels are raised, the chlorine and potassium levels decreased compared to the normal.

DISCUSSION

There are relatively few methods for measuring the physical properties of S.C. and we believe that the techniques used in this investigation provide increased understanding of the horny layer and may help diagnostically. Desquamation is the result of a controlled loss of cohesion between corneocytes and the tests we have employed have been chosen because they either visualize the process of desquamation or measure intracorneal cohesion. The examination of the skin surface replicas from patients with dominant ichthyosis by scanning electron microscopy supports the suggestion that there is an abnormality of desquamation in ichthyotic subjects. The large groups of horn cells which appear to stick to the surface of the specimen perhaps indicate a greater adherence between corneocytes at points where they usually desquamate in normal subjects.

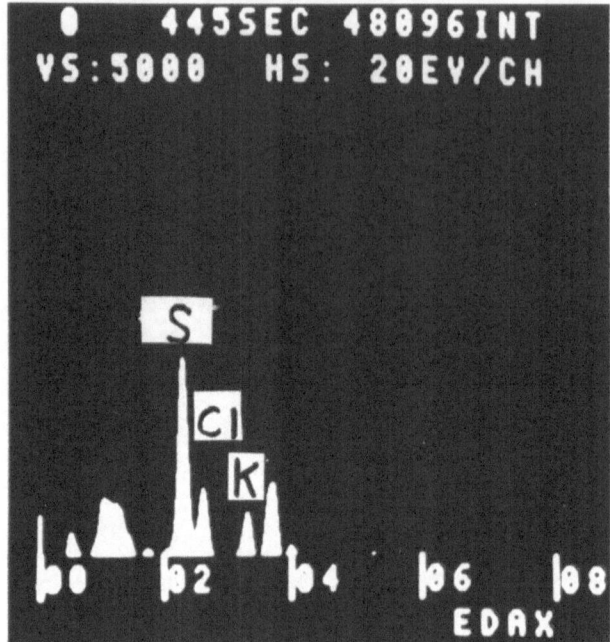

Figure 12.6 An element spectrum of a SSB from a patient with dominant ichthyosis

The concept of greater cohesion in severe ichthyotic stratum corneum is also supported by the cohesograph findings, which are a measure of the vertical breaking strength of horny layer *in vivo*. The areas measured in the surfometer tracings also favours the concept of increased intracorneal cohesion as there is evidence that this measurement reflects the binding forces within the horny layer[2]. The preliminary results of the element distribution in normal and ichthyotic S.C. reveal an interesting difference — but as yet we cannot account for this. We have described the technical detail and other applications of this investigation elsewhere[5].

The physical properties of the stratum corneum are of paramount importance to the function of the S.C. and little attention has been devoted to this important aspect of skin physiology in the past. It is our contention that this area of investigation will become of increasing importance — especially in the evaluation of disorders of keratinization and in the selection of new pharmacological agents which have a therapeutic effect on the S.C.

References

1. Sarkany, I. and Caron, G. (1965). Microtopography of the human skin. *J. Anat.*, **99**, 359

2. Nicholls, S. and Marks, R. (1977). Novel techniques for the estimation of intracorneal cohesion *in vivo*. *Br. J. Dermatol.*, **96,** 595

3. Marks, R. and Dawber, R. P. R. (1971). Skin surface biopsy. An improved technique for examination of the horny layer. *Br. J. Dermatol.*, **84,** 117

4. Marks, R. and Pearse, A. (1975). Surfometry: A method of evaluating the internal structure of the stratum corneum. *Br. J. Dermatol.*, **92,** 1

5. King, C. S., Moore, N., Nicholls, S. and Marks, R. The measurement of percorneal penetration using X-ray microanalysis and scanning electron microscopy (In preparation)

Section 2
Clinical and Genetic Aspects

13
Less Common Scaling Dermatoses

P. FROST

INTRODUCTION

The events which normally transform germinative epithelial cells of the human epidermis into differentiated squamous cells and then into more fully keratinized cells of the stratum corneum (normal keratinization) are poorly understood. Although the morphological consequences of these events are well described for both normal skin and the skin of various pathologic states, the critical biochemical and physiologic parameters which result in a smooth, supple, continuous skin surface or deviation from the more normal condition have not been identified.

A prime reason for focusing attention on the more common ichthyosiform dermatoses and the less common scaling disorders is to attempt to gain insight into important biologic functions associated with the formation of a stratum corneum with normal physical properties and normal barrier function.

Classifications of disorders of keratinization based on genetic and morphologic criteria[1] and even cell kinetic data[2] must be considered tentative, pending understanding of more specific defects which will then identify disorders on a more definitive basis, e.g., Refsum's disease (see Chapters 8, 9).

Yet, for purposes of biologic research and genetic counselling of patients and their families, it is useful to separate various scaling disorders into categories based on whatever distinguishing features are discernible. This is done with the awareness that different genotypes may appear as similar phenotypes and *vice versa*.

The formation of visibly rough and coarse surface scale in various disorders may involve the common feature of decreased *in vivo* water binding capacity so that, under ambient conditions which would normally result in adequate hydration of the stratum corneum, insufficient water is bound. The volume and surface area of the stratum corneum may then become diminished so that it can no longer cover the surface area of the body, and cracks or fissures form (Figure 13.1) as would also occur with relative dryness of other usually hydrated surfaces (Figure 13.2). Forced hydration of the skin surface in these skin disorders can increase the volume and surface area of the stratum corneum and temporarily ameliorate the manifestations of the disorder.

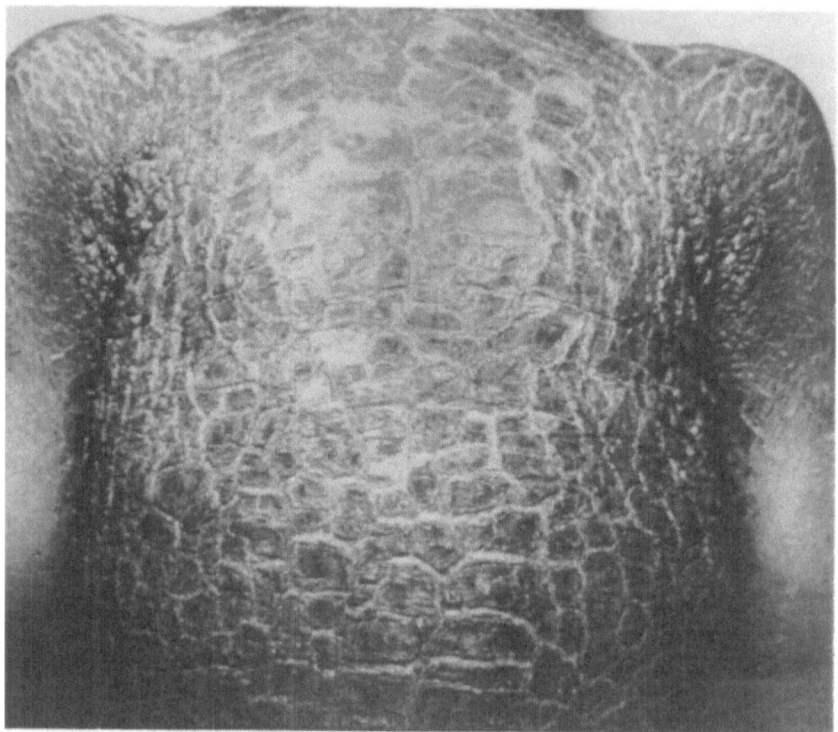

Figure 13.1A   Boy with lamellar ichthyosis showing large flat scales with separations between them

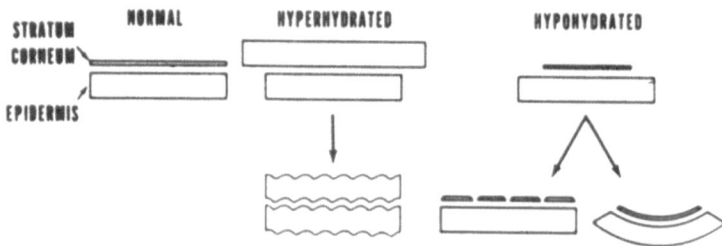

Figure 13.1B   Diagram of scale formation in relation to state of hydration of stratum corneum. Hyperhydrated stratum corneum is thick, as on the palms and soles, after being immersed in water

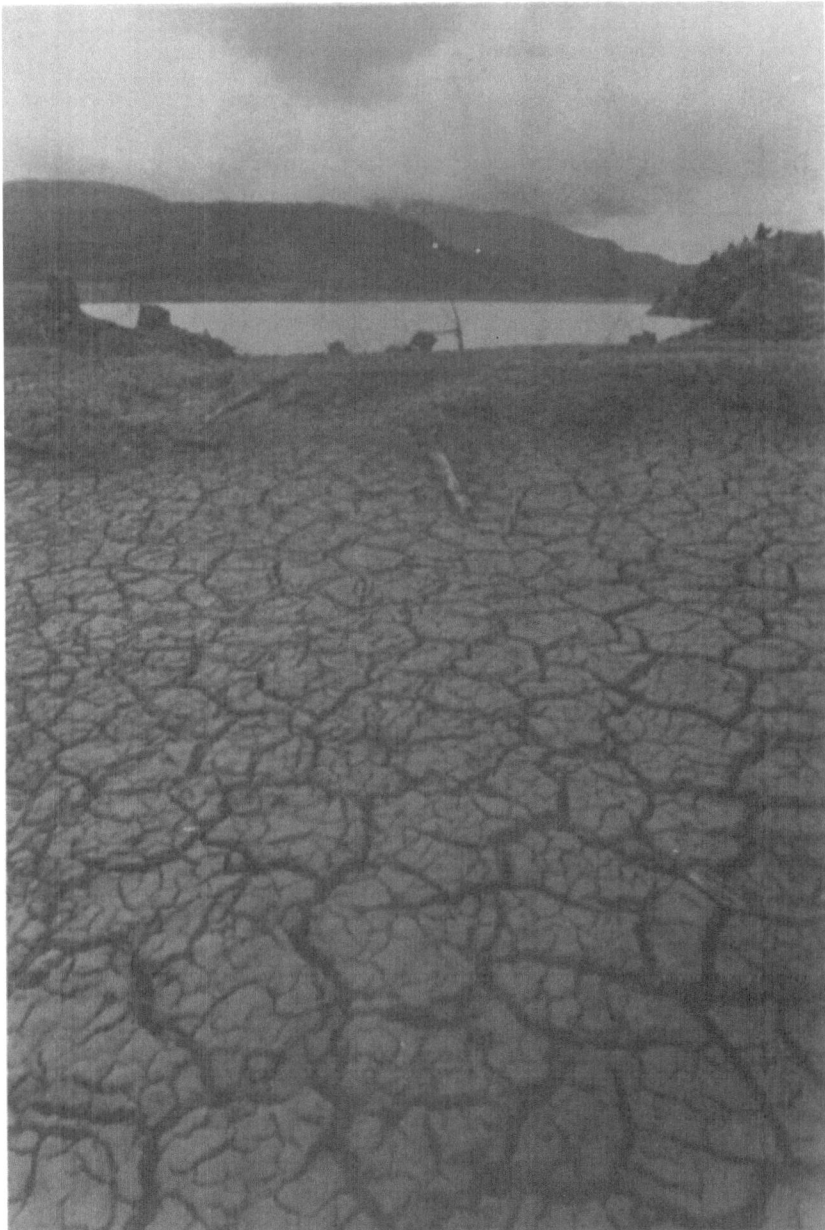

Figure 13.2 Receding water in reservoir behind Merwin Dam. Dehydration of normally moist soil causes shrinking and cracking in a manner analogous to scale formation in human skin. Photograph courtesy Time-Life Inc (Photographer, David Falconer)

Table 13.1 Situations associated with scaling of skin

Drug or abnormal condition	Chemical change
Nicotinic acid	↓ Cholesterol
WY-3547 (A-Butyrophenone)	↓ Cholesterol
Triparanol	↓ Cholesterol
Refsum's disease	Branched fatty acid accumulation
Essential fatty acid deficiency	↓ EFA
Conradi's disease	↓ Serum cholesterol

What chemical abnormalities are associated with these pathophysiologic events? Changes in lipid composition are suggested (Table 13.1) since drugs which decrease the cholesterol content of tissues can cause scaling as a side effect. Low serum cholesterol has been reported in Conradi's disease[3]. Phytanic acid accumulates in Refsum's disease[4]. Essential fatty acid deficiency causes scaling of the skin (Figure 13.3) which clears when essential fatty

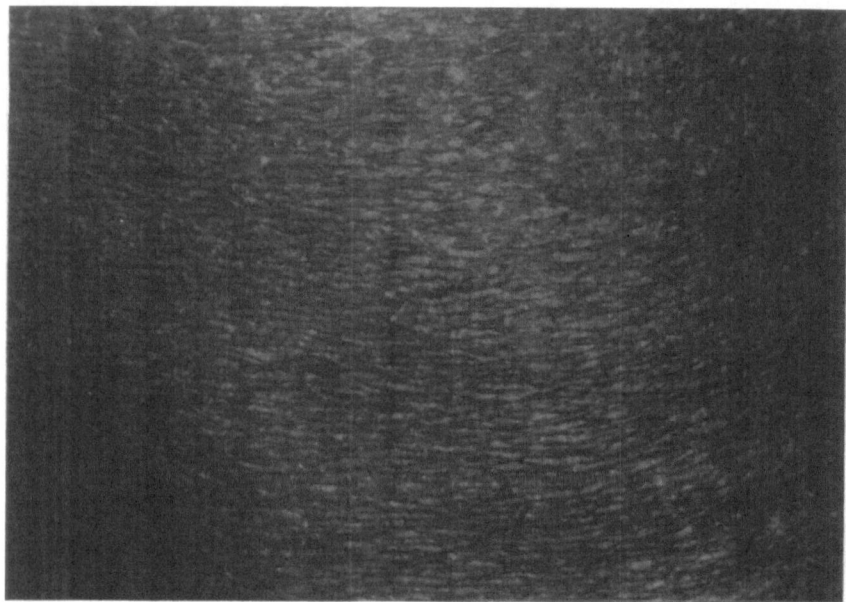

Figure 13.3 Fine scale on abdomen of child with essential fatty acid deficiency resulting from administration of special low fat diet following removal of major part of bowel because of volvulus. Addition of essential fatty acids to diet resulted in complete clearing of scaling

acids are administered[5,6] and, in rats, essential fatty acid deficiency is associated with decreased water binding of the stratum corneum[7]. It is possible that changes of the normal lipid composition of epidermal cells results in cell membranes with diminished ability to retard intracellular water loss, as occurs when normal skin is treated with lipid solvents or detergents[8]. Scaly skin may also have decreased barrier function[9].

Also of interest is the observation that various α-hydroxy acids administered topically to patients with various scaling disorders results in more normal appearing skin (see Chapter 1). Is this a pharmacologic effect? Are the administered α-hydroxy acids replacing deficient similar substrates or end products? It is hoped that close scrutiny of many disorders which have in common abnormal scaling of the skin will help clarify mechanisms of this most complex clinical aberration.

VARIANTS OF MORE COMMON ICHTHYOSIFORM DERMATOSES

Table 13.2 lists the major types of ichthyosis. In each category can be placed patients with unusual forms, with the reservation that a particularly unusual case may not truly be part of a sub-group of that disorder but, rather, either a distinct entity, or a sub-group of another major category.

Lamellar ichthyosis

Erythematous variant

Most patients with lamellar ichthyosis have large, coarse scales that are tan to brown in color (Figure 13.4). Certain patients have more transparent scales with underlying erythema (Figure 13.5). These patients have been under-

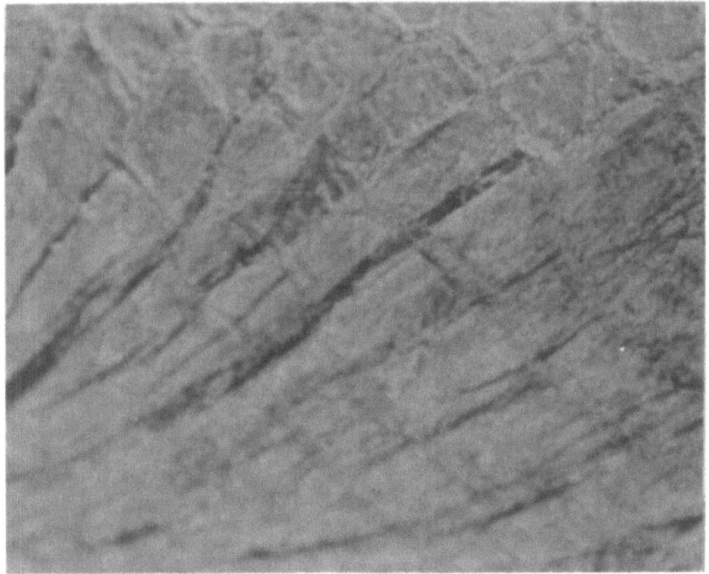

Figure 13.4   Dark coarse scales in patient with ordinary lamellar ichthyosis

Table 13.2 Guide to the major types of ichthyosis

Type	Prevalence	Genetic inheritance	Onset and prognosis	Clinical	Associated features	Pathophysiology and pathology
Lamellar ichthyosis	Rare	Autosomal recessive	Birth; lifelong	Generalized: large scales	Prematurity: ectropion	Increased epidermal kinetics; granular layer normal
Epidermolytic hyperkeratosis	Rare	Autosomal dominant	Birth; lifelong	Generalized; accentuated skin markings; bullae		Increased epidermal kinetics; reticulated granular layer
X-linked ichthyosis	1:6000	X-linked	<1 yr; improvement in summer	Extensor and flexor aspects of extremities; small dark, adherent scales	Asymptomatic corneal deposits in affected males and in female carriers	Hyperkeratosis; normal epidermal kinetics
Ichthyosis vulgaris	1:1000	Autosomal dominant	Three months to teens; may clear with age	Accentuated on extensor aspects of extremities; fine flaky soles; palms and soles markedly involved	Atopy; keratosis pilaris	Normal epidermal kinetics; reduced granular layer
Psoriasiform erythroderma	Rare	Family history of psoriasis	At or near birth; lifelong	Generalized erythema, scaling	Possible ectropion	Histology and epidermal kinetics are like psoriasis
Harlequin fetus	Very rare	Autosomal recessive	Death within two weeks	Generalized, large plaque-like scales	Ectropion; eclabion	Molecular defect in keratin

112

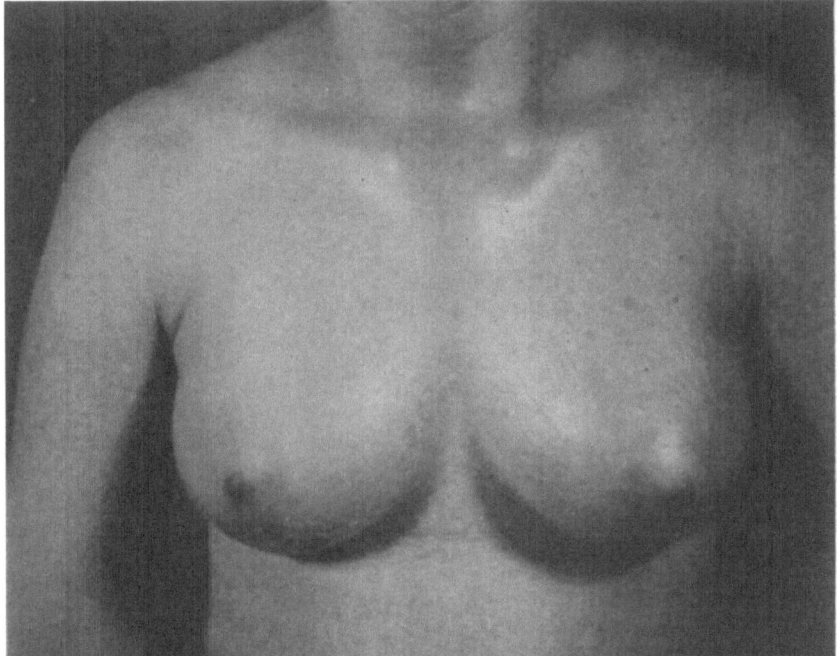

Figure 13.5 A 20-year-old blond girl with variant of lamellar ichthyosis in which scales are more transparent and the skin is slightly erythematous

standably referred to as having non-bullous congenital ichthyosiform erythroderma, although histologic sections of biopsy specimens of their skin are indistinguishable from those from the more typical cases of lamellar ichthyosis. In addition, they resemble patients referred to below as having psoriasiform erythroderma.

Variants with scarring alopecia (and deafness and keratitis)

An unusual manifestation of lamellar ichthyosis is scarring alopecia which probably results from recurring infections of the scalp (Figure 13.6). Other cases have been described with both alopecia, congenital deafness and keratitis[10]. The reported patients occurred sporadically with no family history of similar cases.

Sjögren-Larsson syndrome

Sjögren-Larsson syndrome consists of mental retardation, progressive spastic paralysis, and an ichthyosiform dermatosis that most resembles lamellar ichthyosis grossly and histologically. Like lamellar ichthyosis, it is inherited as an autosomal recessive trait[11].

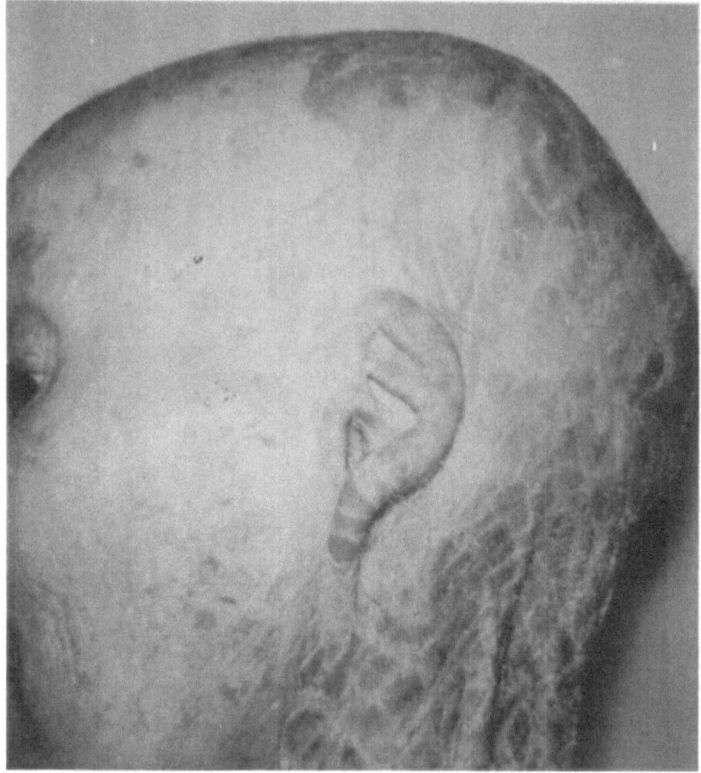

Figure 13.6   Woman with lamellar ichthyosis and scarring alopecia

Harlequin fetus

This is a rare disorder (fewer than 100 reported cases), probably distinct from lamellar ichthyosis, as indicated by X-ray diffraction studies and amino acid analyses of keratin in both conditions[12]. Normal human keratin, upon heating, changes from an α to a cross β pattern, whereas in harlequin fetus, a cross β pattern is present at ambient temperatures. Multiple congenital defects make the condition fatal during the neonatal period. It is listed here since, grossly, the skin resembles an extreme form of collodion baby, a granular layer is present in histologic sections of skin specimens, and it is probably also inherited as an autosomal recessive trait. The skin surface is covered with a thick scaly sheet which is broken by large fissures (Figure 13.7). The external ear is absent or poorly developed.

Epidermolytic hyperkeratosis — localized variants

Although unilateral or other more limited forms of epidermolytic hyper-

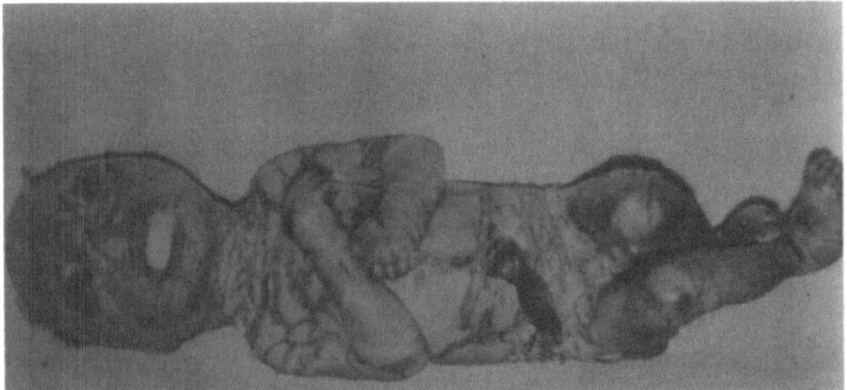

Figure 13.7   Harlequin fetus. Photograph courtesy of Dr. Arnesto Macetelo-Ruiz

keratosis have been described, the most common variant is limited to the palms and soles[13]. Like the generalized form, it is inherited as an autosomal dominant trait.

X-linked ichthyosis

The only variant of this disorder is the minor form that occurs in female hetero-zygote carriers. This consists of mild scaling, particularly of the legs, and corneal densities which do not restrict vision, similar to those occurring in males with the fully expressed form.

Ichthyosis vulgaris

The distinguishing features of ichthyosis vulgaris are autosomal dominant inheritance, mild scaling, and diminished thickness of the granular layer in histologic sections of skin. There is a small group of cases which occur sporadically, appearing to demonstrate either an autosomal recessive pattern of inheritance or a spontaneous mutation. In these patients scaling is severe and extensive so that grossly they resemble patients with lamellar ichthyosis. They are, however, included as variants of ichthyosis vulgaris because of a markedly diminished granular layer thickness.

Psoriasiform erythroderma

This is a disorder in which exfoliative erythroderma is present at birth or occurs during early childhood, and continues into adulthood. Gross and histologic features most closely resemble psoriasis (Figure 13.8). A family history of psoriasis may be present.

Unilateral variant

There are five reported cases of infants who have multiple defects[14]: Unilateral ectromelia, and central nervous system anomalies and a skin disorder similar to that described above in patients with generalized skin involvement, limited to one side of the body. There is also a family history of psoriasis. The unique feature in these cases is that all abnormalities are unilateral (Figure 13.9). The kinetics of epidermal cell proliferation in the psoriasis-like skin are similar to

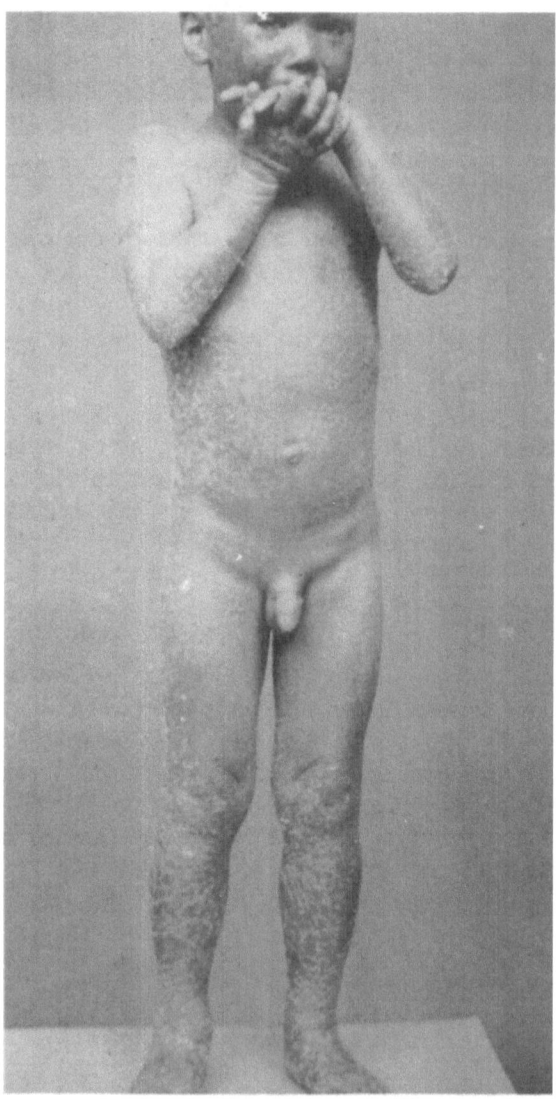

Figure 13.8A Boy with psoriasiform erythroderma. Skin is universally red and scaly

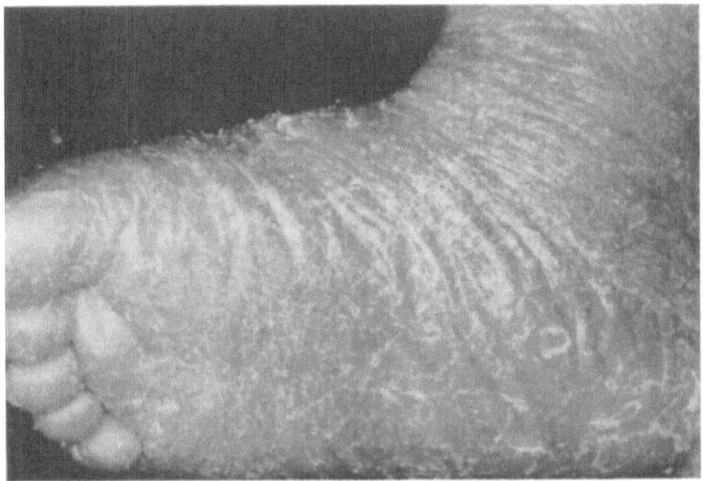

Figure 13.8B   Foot of boy in 13.8A showing micaceous scales

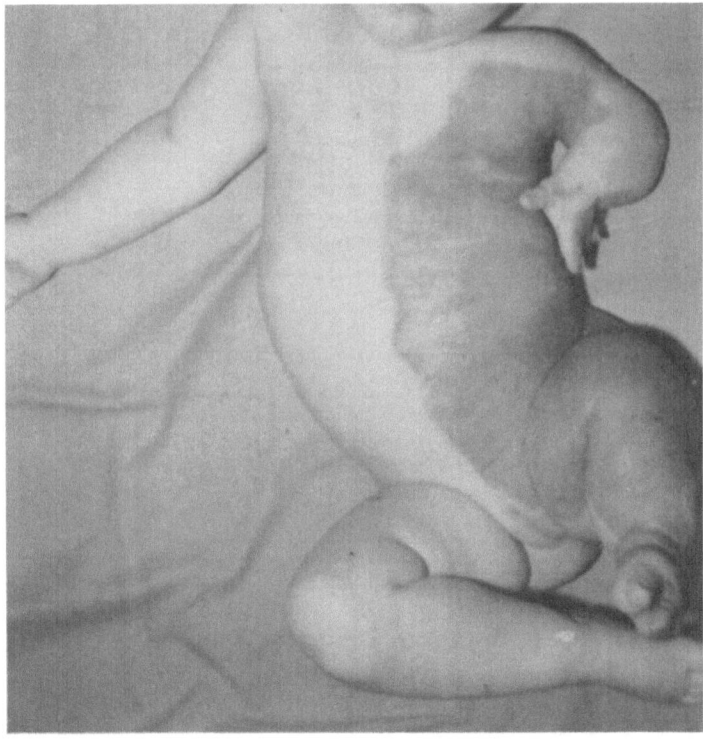

Figure 13.9A   Girl with unilateral ectromelia, limb deformities, and psoriasiform eruption

Summary of Kinetic Studies

KINETICS   OF   SKIN

		LABELED CELLS per cm. S.L.
PATIENT	lt. (normal)	45
	rt. (abnormal)	907
NORMAL SKIN		86
PSORIASIS		959
LAMELLAR ICHTHYOSIS		231
EPIDERMOLYTIC HYPERKERATOSIS		294

Figure 13.9B Summary of labelling experiments utilizing locally injected tritiated thymidine indicating that degree of labelling in patient's skin is similar to that found in psoriasis and normal skin

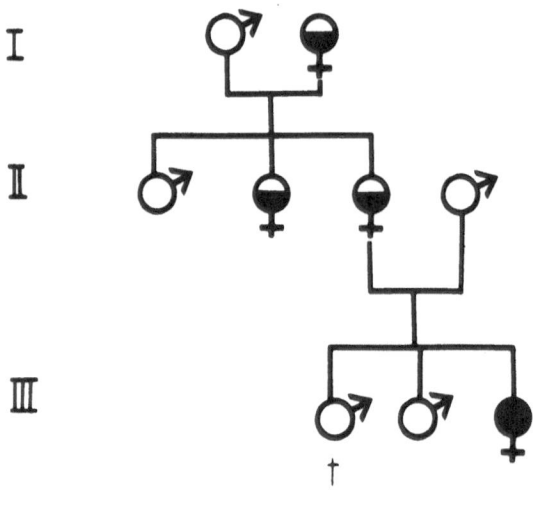

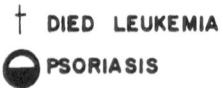

† DIED LEUKEMIA

PSORIASIS

Figure 13.9C   Pedigree of child showing familial occurrence of psoriasis. Propositus is completely blackened

those in ordinary psoriasis; in the normal appearing skin on the opposite side of the body, similar to normal skin in psoriatic patients.

Mal de Meleda

This is the disorder found primarily on the small (40 by 6 kilometer) island of Meleda off the coast of Yugoslavia. Although it has been considered to be a form of keratosis palmaris et plantaris, lesions, which occur shortly after birth, extend to the arms, elbows, knees, and perianal areas[15]. These consist of erythematous, scaly plaques, which may cover the entire palms and soles, but have well demarcated borders. The finger and toe nails may be dystrophic with subungual hyperkeratosis. Histologic sections of skin specimens show hyperkeratosis, parakeratosis, acanthosis, and an inflammatory infiltrate. The pattern of inheritance is unclear because of a high incidence of consanguinity on the island so that autosomal recessive and dominant or multifactorial modes are possibilities.

CONGENITAL TRANSIENT SCALING DISORDERS

Lamellar ichthyosis of the newborn

In this disorder, newborn infants are covered by a collodion membrane. This is transformed into heavy scaling which lasts from a few days[16] to more than a year[17] or two[18] after which there is no further abnormality of the skin apparent. It appears to be inherited as an autosomal recessive trait[19].

Conradi's disease (Chondrodystrophia congenita punctata)

Conradi's disease is a serious multisystem defect usually fatal before age two in which universal erythema and scaling in a whorl and swirl pattern are present at birth. In about three to six months the erythroderma clears but may leave areas of follicular atrophoderma[20] or pseudopelade of the scalp[21]. The most common systemic defects are:

(1) skeletal shortening of humerus and femur
(2) flexion deformities of the elbows and knees with resistance to passive extension
(3) lens opacities and primary optic atrophy
(4) high-arched palate
(5) flat bridged nose
(6) stippled epiphyses on X-rays.

Low serum cholesterol levels were found in two cases[3]; the significance of this finding is not known.

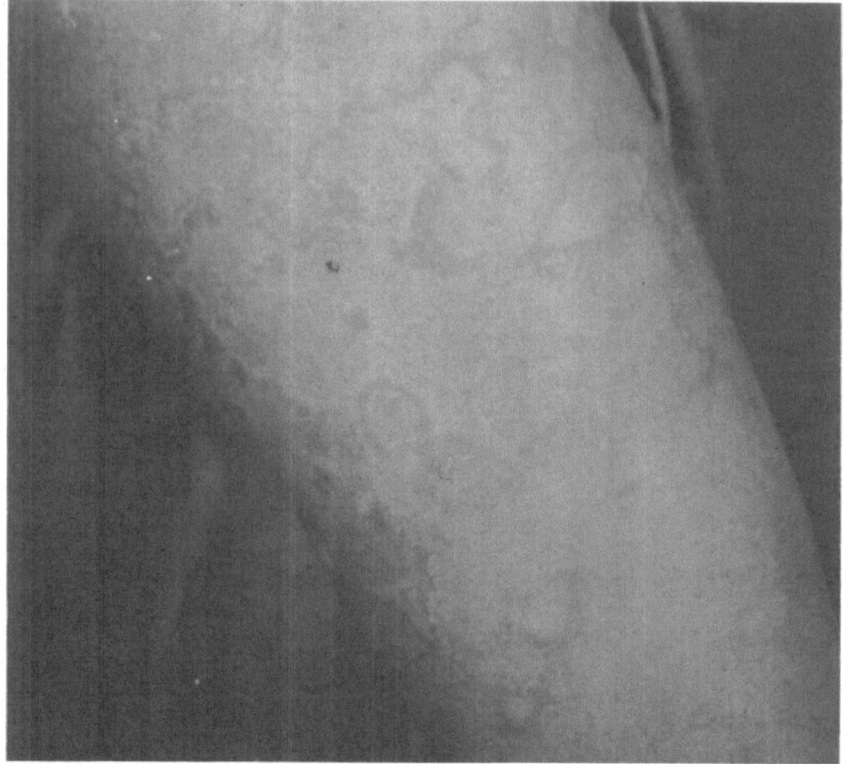

Figure 13.10   Thigh of woman with erythrokeratodermia variabilis

SCALING ASSOCIATED WITH HAIR DEFECTS

Netherton's disease is used to refer to an association of scaling disorders of the skin and hair abnormalities. Although one cannot be sure of the nature of the scaling disorder of Netherton's patients, lamellar ichthyosis is a likely possibility. The hair defect was most likely trichorrhexis invaginata[22]. An association between other hair disorders and other scaling conditions of the skin has also been reported[23]. Ichthyosis linearis circumflexa, along with pila torti, trichorrhexis nodosa, or trichorrhexis invaginata has been described in several patients.

Since the relationship between ichthyosis linearis circumflexa and lamellar or other forms of ichthyosis is not known, it is probably best to reserve the eponym, *Netherton's disease*, only for those patients with lamellar ichthyosis or to avoid using the eponym at all.

GYRATE SCALING DERMATOSES

Erythrokeratodermia variabilis

This is a condition characterized by gyrate erythematous and scaling plaques which remain relatively stationary, and migratory areas of erythema of an urticarial nature (Figure 13.10). It is inherited as an autosomal dominant trait and is present at birth in approximately 30% of cases. In the majority of other cases it occurs during the first year of life.

Little is known about the pathogenesis[24] but the presence of immunoglobulins fixed to the lower layers of the stratum corneum has recently been described[25].

Ichthyosis linearis circumflexa

First described by Comel[26], this disorder begins during infancy with diffuse erythema and scaling which, after a few weeks develops into widespread, migratory, serpiginous and polycyclic areas of scaling with extreme hyperkeratosis of the flexural regions. It is probably inherited as an autosomal recessive trait. It may be associated with hair defects such as pili torti, trichorrhexis nodosa, or trichorrhexis invaginata.

Mixed types

Patients with gyrate scaling dermatoses who do not conform to either of the above categories are occasionally seen. Figure 13.11 depicts an anovulatory woman covered with exuberant hyperkeratotic scale, particularly in the flexural areas of migratory erythema over which the hyperkeratosis is accentuated. Without the gyrate areas of erythema, this patient most closely resembles patients with epidermolytic hyperkeratosis, except that histologic sections of her skin showed only massive hyperkeratosis and acanthosis, but no epidermolytic features.

EPITHELIAL NEVI

This term is used to indicate hyperkeratotic lesions of the skin in which the observable histological changes are limited to hyperkeratosis and slight acanthosis and in which, grossly, a small cobblestone appearance is noted rather than flat scales, as in ichthyosis. The involvement may be generalized, widespread or localized. They may occur as an apparently isolated defect or associated with various systemic anomalies.

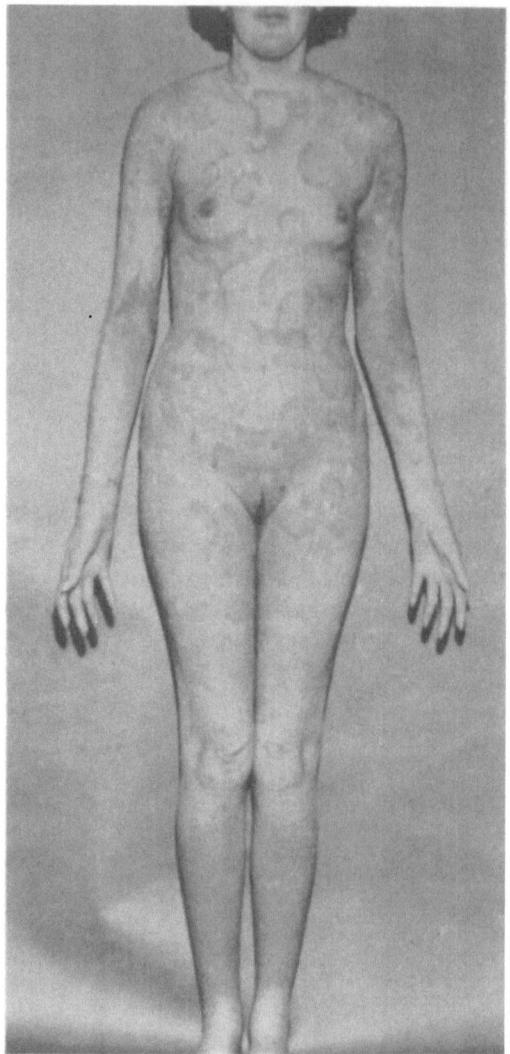

Figure 13.11 Woman with mixed form of gyrate erythema resembling erythrokeratodermia variabilis and epidermolytic hyperkeratosis. Histologic sections of skin specimens showed massive hyperkeratosis, but no epidermolytic features

SCALING OF SKIN ASSOCIATED WITH METABOLIC DISORDERS

Refsum's disease

This disorder, in which neurological defects and scaling are associated with an accumulation of phytanic acid is discussed in Chapter 8.

Hypothyroidism

Mild scaling is associated with hypothyroidism.

Rud's syndrome

This disorder consists of oligophrenia, infantilism, congenital ichthyosis most like lamellar ichthyosis, and possible epilepsy[27]. Patients with these defects who also have a variety of others, have also been described.

Essential fatty acid deficiency

The most characteristic feature of essential fatty acid deficiency in humans is generalized dry, scaly skin with occasional dermatitis of the intertrigenous folds, which clears rapidly upon the administration of linoleic acid or one of its esters or triglycerides[5]. The scaling is fine (Figure 13.4) and histologic sections of skin show hyperkeratosis with a normal appearing granular layer. It is of interest that essential fatty acid deficient rats also develop scaling of the skin[6] and their scale shows deficient water binding capacity[7]. Topical administration of prostaglandin E_2 corrects the scaling in rats[28].

Ichthyosiform scaling and malignancy

Ichthyosiform scaling has been clearly shown to occur in relation to certain cases of lymphoma[29] and other forms of malignancy[30] although no clues as to mechanisms are yet available.

Hansen's Disease

As many as 10% of patients with severe leprosy, particularly of the lepromatous form, may have scaling of the lower extremities and trunk[31]. Again, there is no concept of possible mechanisms.

Inhibitors of lipid synthesis

Nicotinic acid, in large doses[32], the butyrophenones[33], and triparanol[34], all inhibitors of lipid synthesis, may cause, as a side effect, scaling of the skin. Possible mechanisms for this effect are discussed above.

CONCLUSION

Some of the numerous variants of the more common ichthyosiform dermatoses and scaling conditions associated with various metabolic aberrations have been

DEFICIENT OR ABNORMAL LIPIDS

OF STRATUM CORNEUM CELLS

↓

DECREASED WATER BINDING CAPACITY

AND/OR

FAULTY BARRIER AGAINST

WATER LOSS

↓

"DRY" HORNY LAYER

AND SCALE FORMATION

WHEN ATMOSPHERIC CONDITIONS APPROPRIATE

(DRY HEAT, COLD, WIND)

Figure 13.12   Summary of possible relation of skin lipids to scale formation

briefly reviewed. A very general hypothesis of a possible relationship between abnormal or deficient lipids in epidermal cells is presented (Figure 13.12) and it is hoped that, as more specific information is accumulated, a more meaningful understanding of the mechanisms of scale formation and clinical management will follow.

References

1. Wells, R. S. and Kerr, C. B. (1965). Genetic classification of Ichthyosis. *Arch. Dermatol.,* **92,** 1
2. Frost, P., Weinstein, G. D. and Van Scott, E. J. (1966). The ichthyosiform dermatoses. II. Autoradiographic studies of epidermal proliferation. *J. Invest. Dermatol.,* **47,** 561
3. Armaly, M. F. (1957). Ocular involvement in chondrodystrophia calcificans congenita punctata. *A.M.A. Arch. Ophth.,* **57,** 491
4. Baxter, J. H. (1968). Absorption of chlorophyll phytol in normal man and in patients with Refsum's disease. *J. Lipid Res.,* **9,** 636
5. Hansen, A. E., Weise, H. F., Boelsche, A. N., Haggard, M. E., Adam, D. J. and Davis, H. (1963). Role of linoleic acid in infant nutrition. *Pediatrics, Part II, 171*
6. Kingery, F. A. J. and Kellum, R. E. (1965). Essential fatty acid deficiency: Histological changes in the skin of rats. *Arch. Dermatol.,* **91,** 272
7. Sings, E. J. and Vinson, L. J. (1966). The water binding properties of skin. *The Toilet Goods Association,* **46,** 29

8. Middleton, J. D. (1968). The mechanism of water binding in stratum corneum. *Br. J. Dermatol.*, **80,** 437

9. Frost, P., Weinstein, G. D., Bothwell, J. and Wildenauer, R. (1968). The ichthyosiform dermatoses. III. Studies of transepidermal water loss. *Arch. Dermatol.*, **98,** 230

10. Rycroft, R. J. G., Moynahan, E. J. and Wells, R. S. (1976). Atypical ichthyosiform erythroderma, deafness, and keratitis. *Br. J. Dermatol.*, **94,** 211

11. Heijer, A. and Reed, W. B. (1965). Sjögren-Larsson syndrome. *Arch. Dermatol.*, **92,** 545

12. Baden, H. P. and Goldsmith, L. A. (1973). The structural proteins of harlequin fetus: Stratum corneum. *J. Invest. Dermatol.*, **61,** 25

13. Klaus, S., Weinstein, G. D. and Frost, P. (1970). Localized epidermolytic hyperkeratosis. A form of keratoderma of the palms and soles. *Arch. Dermatol.*, **101,** 272

14. Shear, C. S., Nyhan, W. L., Frost, P. and Weinstein, G. D. (1971). Syndrome of unilateral ectromelia, psoriasis and central nervous system anomalies. in *Skin, Hair, and Nails, Birth Defects. Original Article Series.* **7,** No. 8, 197

15. Schnyder, U. W., Franceschetti, A. Th., Ceszarovic, B. and Segedin, J. (1969). Le Maladie de Meleda Autochtone. *Ann de Dermet de Syph.*, **96,** 517

16. Perez, M. (1880). Sclerose general de la peau chez un neaveau-ne. *Rev. Med. Chile*, **68,** 524

17. Bowens, J. T., (1895). The epitricheal layer of the epidermis and its relationship to ichthyosis congenita. *J. Cutan. Genitourin Dis.*, **13,** 485

18. Carini, A. (1895). Di una ferma attenuata della cosidetta ittosi sebacea (ittosi lamellare). *G. Ital. Mal Vener.*, **30,** 82

19. Reed, W. B., Herwick, R. P., Harville, D., Porter, P. S. and Conant, M. (1972). Lamellar ichthyosis of the newborn. *Arch. Dermatol.*, **105,** 394

20. Bodian, E. L. (1966). Skin manifestations of Conradi's disease. *Arch. Dermatol.*, **94,** 743

21. Comings, D. E., Papazian, C. and Schoene, H. R., (1968). Conradi's disease, *J. Pediat.*, **72,** 63

22. Netherton, E. W. (1958). A unique case of trichorrhexis nodosa 'bamboo hairs'. *Arch. Dermatol.*, **78,** 483

23. Hurwitz, S., Kirsch, N. and McGuire, J. (1971). Reevaluation of ichthyosis and hair shaft abnormalities. *Arch. Dermatol.*, **103,** 266

24. Brown, J. and Kierland, R. R. (1966). Erythrokeratodermia variabilis. *Arch. Dermatol.*, **93,** 194

25. Gewertzman, G. Personal communication

26. Comel, M. (1949). Ichthyosis linearis circumflexa. *Dermatologica*, **98,** 133

27. Rud, E. (1929). Et tilfaelded of hypogenitalisme (eunochodismus feminus) med partiel gigantisme og ichthyosis. *Hospitalitidende*, **72,** 426

28. Ziboh, V. A. and Hsia, S. L. (1972). Effects of prostaglandin E_2 on rat skin: Inhibition of sterol ester biosynthesis and clearing of scaling lesions in essential fatty acid deficiency. *J. Lipid Res.*, **13,** 458

29. Frost, P. and Shalhub, S. (1976). Ichthyosiform scaling in association with lymphoma. *South. Med. J.*, **69,** 504

30. Flint, G. L., Flam, M. and Soter, N. A. (1975). Acquired ichthyosis. A sign of a non-lymphoproliferative malignant disorder. *Arch. Dermatol.*, **111,** 1446

31. Schulz, R. J. (1965). Ichthyosiform conditions occurring in Leprosy. *Br. J. Dermatol.*, **77,** 151

32. Parsons, W. B. and Flinn, J. H. (1959). Reduction of serum cholesterol levels and beta-lipoprotein levels by nicotinic acid. *Arch. Int. Med.*, **103,** 123

33. Simpson, G. M. and Cranswick, E. H. (1964). Cutaneous effects of a new butyrophenone drug. *Clin. Pharmacol. Ther.*, **5,** 310

34. Winkelmann, R. K., Perry, H. O. and Achor, R. W. (1963). Cutaneous syndromes produced as side effects of triparanol therapy. *Arch. Dermatol.*, **87,** 372

14
Genetic Heterogeneity in the Ichthyoses

P. S. HARPER

INTRODUCTION

The inherited nature of many of the ichthyotic disorders has been clear since their original clinical recognition, and the early genetic studies of Cockayne[1] and others provided some of the most conclusive examples of simple Mendelian inheritance in human disease. During subsequent years an almost universal finding in genetic disorders has been the phenomenon of genetic heterogeneity; this has proved particularly widespread in the ichthyoses, so that a considerable number of distinct inherited disorders can now be recognized, in addition to others whose separate identity is less secure. The major forms are summarized in Table 14.1. The accurate recognition of this heterogeneity is fundamental to our understanding of the underlying molecular basis of this group of conditions, particularly as their investigation is now moving from a purely descriptive phase to a study of their biochemical nature. In this paper the ways in which genetic heterogeneity may be suspected and established are outlined, together with the consequences resulting from it.

THE RECOGNITION OF HETEROGENEITY

The traditional, and still the fundamental method of approach to hetero-geneity is to analyse the clinical features of the disorders in question in relation to the pattern of inheritance observed in families. This may produce obvious differences between forms which leave no doubt that they are clinically and genetically distinct. Thus congenital 'lamellar' ichthyosis is clearly a different entity from ichthyosis vulgaris occurring in adult life, and the finding that in the former the inheritance is autosomal recessive, with multiple affected

127

Table 14.1   The inherited ichthyosis — clinical and genetic classification

Disorder	Inheritance
Ichthyosis without syndromal association	
Congenital ichthyosis	
(a) Lamellar ichthyosis (collodion baby)	Autosomal recessive
(b) Harlequin fetus (lethal)	Autosomal recessive
Ichthyosis hystrix	Autosomal dominant
Ichthyosis vulgaris	Autosomal dominant
X-linked ichthyosis	X-linked recessive
Syndromes associated with ichthyosis	
Refsum syndrome	Autosomal recessive
Ichthyosis with mental retardation and spastic tetraplegia.	
(Sjögren-Larsson syndrome)	Autosomal recessive
Ichthyosis with male hypogonadism	X-linked recessive
Conradi's syndrome (chondrodysplasia punctata)	Autosomal dominant or autosomal recessive
Ichthyosiform erythroderma with deafness	Autosomal recessive
Ichthyosiform erythroderma with unilateral limb defects	Autosomal recessive
Ichthyosis congenita with cataract	Autosomal recessive
Ichthyosis with mental retardation and hypogonadism	
(Rud's syndrome)	Autosomal recessive

sibs born to healthy parents, while in the latter disorder autosomal dominant inheritance is the rule, confirms the clinical impression that the two entities are fundamentally different. Nevertheless, even in such an apparently obvious situation this conclusion should not be reached without considering other alternatives: the possibility that the congenital form represents the homozygous state for the adult form can readily be excluded by the normality of the parents, while other forms of relationship are made unlikely by the fact that no increase in one of the types is seen in families affected by the other.

A less obvious, but now well established example of the combined use of clinical and genetic criteria is the separation of the X-linked and autosomal dominant forms of adult ichthyosis. Although individual pedigrees showing X-linked recessive inheritance had been recognized by Cockayne[1] and even previously by Sedgwick[2], Kerr and Wells[3] were the first to demonstrate that the X-linked form was both clinically and genetically distinct, and that it accounted for over a quarter of cases of ichthyosis in males previously regarded as having ichthyosis vulgaris. By discounting those families in which mode of inheritance was not clear and comparing the clinical features of definitely X-linked families with those showing definitely autosomal dominant inheritance, the X-linked form was shown to be associated with a number of distinctive features, including onset in the early months of life, generally greater severity and larger scale size, and progressive involvement of the trunk[4]. Corneal opacities have also been shown to occur in the X-linked form only[5].

X-linkage offers several unique features that can be utilized to test whether this mode of inheritance is in fact operating. Because of the phenomenon of X-chromosome inactivation in females[6] a variable degree of clinical abnormality is usually seen in heterozygous female carriers, and this is the case with X-linked ichthyosis. Mild scaling of the limbs may occur[7], as may the corneal opacities characteristic of the hemizygous males[5]. The relatively benign nature of the disorder frequently results in affected males reproducing, all of whose daughters must be carriers while their sons should all be unaffected; this again was borne out by the genetic studies of Kerr and Wells[3]. Finally these authors were able in their study to prove linkage between the loci for X-linked ichthyosis and the X_g blood group, with a recombination fraction of around 0.23; this genetic marker is now known also to be linked to the locus for Fabry's disease[8].

Genetic linkage studies provide a potentially valuable method of recognizing genetic heterogeneity in autosomal as well as in X-linked disorders, and although the mapping of the human genome is still at an early stage, there have been rapid advances during the past few years[9]. The non-lethal nature and accurate documentation of many dermatological disorders has allowed linkage analysis from family data to be undertaken for a number of relatively rare conditions: thus the nail-patella syndrome has been known for some time to be linked to the ABO blood group system[10] which has now been located on chromosome 9. Similarly one form of epidermolysis bullosa is linked to the locus for the enzyme glutamate — pyruvate transaminase[11], while the rare form of sclerotylosis with malignant skin change shows close linkage with the MN blood group system[12,13] and which may be located on chromosome 2[14]. This last example shows how linkage data can establish non-allelism, since the common form of palmo-plantar hyperkeratosis (tylosis) does not show linkage with the MN system. The two conditions are thus not just different alleles at the same locus, but are controlled by different loci, with a different fundamental biochemical basis likely.

The development of cell hybridization techniques[15,16] has greatly extended the information on genetic linkage obtainable by family studies, and has resulted in the assignment of numerous biochemical markers to specific chromosomes. Since with few exceptions we do not yet understand disorders of keratinization in enzymatic terms, and have no abnormalities reliably identifiable in cultured cells, this approach has not yet been exploited directly in the ichthyoses and related disorders, but is likely to prove extremely valuable once primary biochemical abnormalities are found.

An example of the power of the cell hybridization approach in resolving genetic heterogeneity can be seen in recent work on xeroderma pigmentosum. Clinical and genetic studies originally suggested this to be a single genetic disorder (possibly two if the DeSanctis–Cacchione form with neurological abnormalities is included). Once the defect in repair of nucleic acid was identified[17] it became clear that some clinically indistinguishable cases of the disease failed to show the biochemical abnormalities[18] and that heterogeneity was likely. Studies on hybrid cells have shown that correction of the cellular defect occurs when normal and defective cells are fused, and that fusion between affected cells from different patients may also produce correction in some instances[19]. From such studies it is clear that at least four biochemically distinct types of Xeroderma pigmentosum exist, with cells from one type able to correct the different abnormality present in another type; within a group correction does not occur. There is no reason why the ichthyoses may not prove to be equally heterogeneous once sufficient biochemical understanding has been achieved to approach them in this way.

Heterogeneity may on occasion be demonstrated by simple family studies, when marriages occur between affected parents. Although such situations have not been recorded for the ichthyoses, oculocutaneous albinism provides a striking example: here two affected parents have produced normal children[20], a situation impossible if both parents had the same allelic form of this recessively inherited condition. This genetic evidence for non-allelic heterogeneity has subsequently been confirmed by the finding of biochemical differences[21], one parent showing the total pigmentary defect associated with absent tyrosinase, while a slight degree of pigmentation and normal tyrosinase activity was present in the other parent.

Pathological studies of the skin have been increasingly used to differentiate the inherited ichthyoses. In addition to classical histology and histochemistry, electron microscopy has been particularly informative[22]. Although such differences may at times reflect secondary factors rather than implying a fundamentally different basis, they provide valuable evidence that can be correlated with clinical and genetic data, and which may confirm or refute heterogeneity postulated on these grounds. Thus autosomal dominant ichthyosis vulgaris and X-linked ichthyosis demonstrate clear differences which support their clinical and genetic distinction. A thin or absent granular cell layer of the epidermis is characteristic of the former, with small and abnormal keratohyalin granules seen on electron-microscopy; in the X-linked form the granular layer is entirely normal on light microscopy, while the electron microscope shows reduced numbers of keratinosomes but normal keratohyalin production[22].

SYNDROMES AND EXPERIMENTAL FORMS OF ICHTHYOSIS

The existence of specific syndromes of which ichthyosis forms a part, provides a particularly valuable opportunity both for recognizing heterogeneity and for understanding the underlying pathogenesis. Some of these syndromes are summarized in Table 14.1. In some such syndromes the skin changes may not themselves be readily distinguishable on clinical and histological grounds from the isolated forms of ichthyosis, but they provide the possibility of finding a common causative factor that can be implicated in both the ichthyosis and the other features of the syndrome. Refsum's syndrome, in which phytanic acid and other fatty acids accumulate as a consequence of deficiency of phytanic acid oxidase, provides an excellent example, being not only a specific entity within the group of inherited ichthyoses but also showing one of the underlying factors, disordered fatty acid metabolism, which may be involved in the production of other forms of the ichthyoses. As with other inborn errors of metabolism, the identification of the precise nature of the enzymatic defect has allowed the potential preclinical and even prenatal detection of the disorder in a way that is usually impossible when clinical and histological criteria have to be relied upon alone.

Careful study of the skin lesions in the syndromes associated with keratinization disorders may show unexpectedly specific changes in the skin itself; these may be ultrastructural or biochemical as in Refsum's syndrome (see Chapters 8, 9), or mainly clinical. Thus in the families with palmoplantar hyperkeratosis associated with oesophageal cancer[23,24] onset of the hyperkeratosis was found to be relatively late in childhood in comparison with the common form unassociated with malignancy, in which most families show onset in the first months of life[25].

No comparable primary biochemical abnormality to that of Refsum's syndrome has so far been found for the other syndromes associated with ichthyosis, but a strong presumption for an enzymatic basis can be made for those showing recessive inheritance, such as the Sjögren-Larsson syndrome and Rud's syndrome. The Sjögren-Larsson syndrome, where ichthyosis is associated with mental retardation and a variable degree of spastic neurological degeneration, provides an important demonstration of the value of isolated communities in defining rare syndromes, since all of the original 28 cases could be shown to have originated from the same common ancestor in Northern Sweden, leaving no doubt that the gene being studied was indeed the same in each instance[26]. In some disorders, such as Conradi's syndrome, where ichthyotic skin changes are associated with punctate calcification and dysplasia of the bony epiphyses, cataract, and in some cases mental retardation, the existence of two distinct forms of inheritance is an indication of genetic heterogeneity within the syndrome itself[27]. Conradi's syndrome also illustrates a further complication for which the investigator must be alert — the existence of phenocopies. Instances have now been recorded in which the syndrome appears not to have a genetic basis, but to have resulted from maternal warfarin ingestion in early pregnancy[28].

No clear distinction is at present possible between such teratogenic cases and the implications are considerable for genetic counselling. As yet the mechanism of action of the drug is unknown, but it is possible that it will provide a clue to the biochemical defect in the genetic forms of this syndrome.

A somewhat similar situation is seen in the ichthyosis which may result from the administration of hypocholesterolaemic drugs such as triparanol and diazacholesterol[29]. Other complications of these agents include cataract and myotonia, and the syndrome they produce may closely resemble the genetically determined myotonic dystrophy, though this disorder does not share the ichthyosis. In this case as with warfarin and Conradi's syndrome, the drug-induced disorder may point to possible causative factors in the genetic condition, the likely mechanism here being alteration in the lipid composition of cell membranes of various tissues[30].

The existence of potential drug models for the inherited ichthyosis raises the question of the validity of data from inherited ichthyosis in experimental animals. Thus one form of ichthyosis (ic) in the mouse is determined by an autosomal recessive form of inheritance[31], while another such mutant ('scurfy') is X-linked. Caution is clearly indicated before morphological or biochemical data on such animal models can be equated with changes in the human ichthyoses, but it should be noted that the X chromosome has been remarkably conservative throughout mammalian evolution, with numerous examples known of homologous conditions being X-linked in widely different species[32]. Thus an X-linked ichthyosis mutant might throw light on the underlying defect in human X-linked ichthyosis in a way which is less likely for autosomally inherited animal models.

THE SIGNIFICANCE OF HETEROGENEITY

Once genetic heterogeneity has been established within a disorder previously considered to be a single entity, the question arises as to whether the different forms are controlled by alleles at the same genetic locus, or whether separate loci are involved. This question is not only of interest to the geneticist but is essential to answer if the disorders are to be fully understood in biochemical terms, since with alleles at the same locus the same disordered enzyme or other protein is to be expected, with differently altered activity or other properties resulting from the different nature of the mutation that it has undergone. By contrast, if the forms are non-allelic, the experience of all inborn errors of metabolism so far identified shows that a fundamentally different primary defect is likely, although the deficient products may be involved in the same metabolic pathway.

It is essential that biochemical and other studies take into account the significance of both allelic and non-allelic heterogeneity in the interpretation of results. Thus the finding of a similar enzymatic abnormality in two forms of ichthyosis known not to be allelic (e.g. autosomal dominant and X-linked ichthyosis) would indicate that the abnormality was not the primary bio-chemical defect, while for allelic forms the same primary defect is to be expected. Most important of all is the danger of missing or misinterpreting a significant abnormality by the lumping together of cases which are known to be heterogeneous on the basis of the different inheritance or other evidence. Even if such data have to be combined for purposes of statistical analysis, they should always be presented in a form allowing separate study in case significant differences are documented subsequently.

From what has been said so far it may seem that the genetic approach is likely to multiply the degree of heterogeneity recognized on clinical grounds to a confusing extent. On occasion this may be true, though in the ichthyoses the majority of splitting into separate groups has so far resulted from clinical differentiation. It is important to realize, however, that genetic studies can equally disprove heterogeneity postulated on clinical and pathological grounds. Thus family studies may show a wide range of expression of a disorder in a single family, where a single abnormal gene is known to be acting, that might clinically have been classed as two or more separate entities. The ichthyoses do not provide a ready example of this, but the author's work on myotonic dystrophy[33,34] showed that the congenital and adult forms of this disease, with striking clinical differences which had led them to be classed as separate disorders, in fact always occurred within the same families, so that genetic heterogeneity was most unlikely. The ichthyoses themselves show one disorder whose unique nature did not stand the test of rigorous genetic study. The occurrence of ichthyosis hystrix gravior in males of the Lambert family was for many years considered to be an example of inheritance on the human Y chromosome, with male to male transmission through numerous generations. The work of Penrose and Stern[35] conclusively disproved this by finding examples of unaffected males and affected females in the family, which had previously been suppressed to fit in with the popular conception of the limitation of the condition to males.

The use of cell culture studies has also disproved as well as established heterogeneity in some cases. Thus studies of cross-correction of the metabolic abnormality in cells from patients with mucopolysaccharidoses established a number of separate groups corresponding in general with recognized clinical criteria[36]. However two disorders, the Hurler (type I) and Scheie (type V) forms of mucopolysaccharidosis, failed to show any cross correction, despite considerable phenotypic differences. The previously unexpected prediction that these two disorders had the same fundamental defect was confirmed by the finding of absent α-L-iduronidase in both[37].

The relatively high frequency of autosomal dominant ichthyosis vulgaris raises some special problems regarding possible heterogeneity, as well as regarding the possible underlying reasons for its commonness. The accepted incidence of around 1 in 2000 births may result in part from the lack of selection against the gene owing to its relatively mild phenotypic effects. This does not fully explain the reason for the gene reaching such a high frequency in the first instance, and it would seem possible that some direct or indirect selective advantage of the gene may have existed in the past which favoured its retention. If on the other hand autosomal dominant ichthyosis were to be shown to be itself heterogeneous, with a number of genes determining it, each individually less common, then there would be no need to postulate such mechanisms for the maintenance of a high gene frequency. At present no evidence exists to resolve this point, but the offspring of marriages between two affected individuals would be expected to be sufficiently frequent to provide evidence.

Should the homozygous state for this disorder exist it would be expected by analogy with other autosomal dominant conditions (e.g. hereditary haemorrhagic telangiectasia) to be much more severe than the heterozygous form, and possibly lethal. So far no definite reports of such individuals have appeared, despite the mention of individuals with two affected parents[7]. A deficiency of homozygotes might suggest that autosomal dominant ichthyosis is indeed genetically heterogeneous and that the affected parents had different forms of the disorder, a situation comparable to that discussed earlier for oculo-cutaneous albinism. A further point of potential importance is that the study of homozygotes, if they do exist, might prove more fruitful in elucidating the biochemical basis than study of heterozygotes has been so far. On general principles it would be expected for it to be easier to identify complete or near complete absence of the primary enzyme or other protein determined by the gene, than to recognize a 50% reduction in the heterozygote. A practical illustration of this is seen in familial hypercholesteraemia (type II hyper-lipoproteinaemia) in which the underlying enzymatic deficiency of HMG CoA reductase was only recognized when the rare homozygotes for the disorder were studied[38] and which proved to be the clue for understanding of the lipid disorder in the heterozygote.

CONCLUSIONS

It can be concluded that heterogeneity in the group of inherited ichthyoses is already marked, and that it is likely to increase as the result of greater understanding of the underlying basis of these disorders. The combined use of clinical, genetic and other investigative techniques should serve to ensure that this heterogeneity is accurately recognized, and will aid in our understanding not only of the ichthyotic disorders, but of the normal processes of keratinization.

References

1. Cockayne, E. A. (1933). *Inherited Abnormalities of the Skin and its Appendages* (London: Oxford University Press)
2. Sedgewick, W. (1863). On the influence of sex in hereditary disease, *British and Foreign Medical-Chirurgical Review*, **31**, 445
3. Kerr, C. B. and Wells, R. S. (1965). Sex linked ichthyosis. *Ann. Hum. Genet.*, **29**, 33
4. Wells, R. S. and Kerr, C. B. (1966). The histology of ichthyosis. *J. Invest. Dermatol.*, **46**, 530
5. Sever, R., Frost, P. and Weinstein, G. D. (1968). Eye changes in ichthyosis. *J. Amer. Med. Ass.*, **206**, 2283
6. Lyon, M. (1961). Gene action in the X chromosome of the mouse (Mus musculus L.) *Nature* (London), **190**, 372

7. Frost, P. (1973). Ichthyosiform dermatoses. *J. Invest. Dermatol.*, **60**, 541

8. Johnston, A. W., Frost, P., Spaeth, G. Z. and Renwick, J. H. (1969). Linkage relationships of the angiokeratoma (Fabry) locus. *Ann. Hum. Genet.*, **32**, 369

9. Bergsma, D. (1976). Ed. Human Gene Mapping 3. (Basel: Karger)

10. Renwick, J. H. and Lawler, S. D. (1955). Genetical linkage between the ABO and nail-patella loci. *Ann. Hum. Genet.*, **19**, 312

11. Olaisen, B. and Gedde-Dahl, T. (1973). GPT-epidermolysis bullosa simplex (EBS Ogna) linkage in man. *Hum. Hered.*, **23**, 189

12. Mennecier, M. (1967). Individualisation d'une nouvelle entité: la génodermatose scléro-atrophiante et kératodermique des extrémités fréquemment dégénérative. Etude clinique et génetique (possibilité de linkage avec le system MNSS). M.D. Thesis, U. de Lille

13. Huriez, C., Deminatti, M., Agache, P. and Mennecier, M. (1968). Une guenodysplasie non encore individualisés: la génodermatose scléro-atrophiante et kératodermique des extrémités fréquemment dégénérative. *Sem. Hop. (Paris)*, **44**, 481

14. German, J. and Chaganti, R. S. K. (1973). Mapping human autosomes: assignment of the MN locus to a specific segment in the long arm of chromosome No. 2. *Science*, **182**, 1261

15. Harris, H. and Watkins, J. F. (1965). Hybrid cells derived from mouse and man: artificial heterokaryons of mammalian cells from different species. *Nature* (London), **205**, 640

16. Ephrussi, B. (1972). *Hybridisation of Somatic Cells* (New Jersey: Princeton University Press)

17. Cleaver, J. E. (1968). Defective repair application of DNA in xeroderma pigmentosum. *Nature (London)*, **218**, 652

18. Cleaver J. E. (1972). Xeroderma pigmentosum: variants with normal DNA repair and normal sensitivity to U.V. light. *J. Invest. Dermatol.*, **58**, 124

19. Robbins, J. C., Kraemer, K. H. Lutzner, M., Festoff, B. W. and Coon, H. G. (1974). Xeroderma pigmentosum: an inherited disease with sun sensitivity, multiple cutaneous neoplasms and abnormal DNA repair. *Ann. Int. Med.*, **80**, 221

20. Trevor-Roper, P. D. (1952). Marriage of two complete albinos with normally pigmented offspring. *Br. J. Ophthalmol.*, **36**, 107

21. Witkop, C. J., Nance, W., Rawls, R. and White, J. (1970). Autosomal recessive oculo-cutaneous albinism in man: evidence for genetic heterogeneity. *Am. J. Hum. Genet.*, **22**, 55

22. Anton-Lamprecht, I. and Schnyder, U. W. (1974). Ultrastructure of inborn errors of keratinisation. VI. Inherited ichthyoses — a model system for heterogeneities in keratinisation disturbances. *Arch. Dermatol. Forsch.*, **250**, 207

23. Howel-Evans, A. W., McConnell, R. B., Clarke, C. A. and Sheppard, P. M. (1958). Carcinoma of the oesophagus with keratosis palmaris et plantaris (tylosis): a study of two families. *Q. J. Med.*, **27**, 413

24. Harper, P. S., Harper, R. M. J. and Howel-Evans, A. W. (1970). Carcinoma of the oesophagus with tylosis. *Q. J. Med.*, **39**, 317

25. Harper, P. S. (1971). Genetic heterogeneity in hyperkeratosis palmaris et plantaris. *Birth Defects original articles series*, **7**, 50

26. Sjögren, T., and Larsson, T. (1957). Oligophrenia in combination with congenital ichthyosis and spastic disorders. A clinical and genetic study. *Acta Psychiatr. Neurol. Scand.*, **32** (Suppl. 113), 1

27. Spranger, J. W., Opitz, J. M. and Bidder, U. (1971). Heterogeneity of chondrodysplasia punctata. *Humangenetik*, **11**, 190

28. Pauli, R. M., Madden, J. D., Kranzler, K. J., Culpepper, W. and Port, R. (1976). Warfarin therapy initiated during pregnancy and phenotypic chondrodysplasia punctata. *J. Ped.*, **88**, 506

29. Achor, R. W. P., Winkelmann, R. K. and Perry, H. O. (1961). Cutaneous side effects from the use of Triparanol (Mer 29): Preliminary data on ichthyosis and loss of hair. *Proc. Mayo Clin.*, **36**, 217

30. Peter, J. B., Dromgoole, S. H. and Campion, D. S. (1975). Experimental myotonia and hypocholesterolemic agents. *Exp. Neurol.*, **49**, 115

31. Green, M. C., Alpert, B. N. and Mayer, T. C. (1974). The site of action of the ichthyosis locus (i.e.) in the mouse, as determined by dermal epidermal recombinations. *J. Embryol. Exp. Morphol.*, **32**, 715

32. Ohno, S. (1967). *Sex Chromosomes and Sex-Linked Genes* (Berlin: Springer)

33. Harper, P. S. (1973). Presymptomatic detection and genetic counselling in myotonic dystrophy. *Clin. Genet.*, **4**, 134

34. Harper, P. S. (1975). Congenital myotonic dystrophy in Britain. II. Genetic aspects. *Arch. Dis. Child.*, **50**, 514

35. Penrose, L. S. and Stern, C. (1958). Reconsideration of the Lambert pedigree (ichthyosis hystrix gravior). *Ann. Hum. Genet.*, **22**, 258

36. Neufeld, E. F. and Cantz, M. J. (1971). Corrective factors for inborn errors of mucopolysaccharide metabolism. *Ann. N.Y. Acad. Sci.*, **179**, 580

37. Bach, G., Friedman, R., Weissmann, B. and Neufeld, E. F. (1972). The defect in the Hurler and Scheie syndromes: deficiency of L-iduronidase. *Proc. Nat. Acad. Sci. U.S.A.*, **69**, 2048

38. Brown, M. S. and Goldstein, J. L. (1974). Familial hypercholesterolemia: defective binding of lipoproteins to cultured fibroblasts associated with impaired regulation of 3-hydroxy-3-methylglutaryl coenzyme A reductase activity. *Proc. Nat. Acad. Sci.*, **71**, 788

15
Inherited Ichthyosiform Dermatoses in Infants and Children

F. GIANOTTI

INTRODUCTION

Clinical features of the inherited ichthyosiform dermatoses have been known since ancient times, but their classification has been substantially modified since their mode of inheritance, histopathology, ultrastructure and biology have been investigated. Excellent classifications have recently been published[1-4]. The one proposed by us (see Tables 15.1, 2 and 3) depends on age of onset, mode of inheritance, and clinical and histological features. These can be recognised by every dermatologist and can therefore be helpful in making a correct diagnosis. In this way, we can answer the anxious parents who want to know everything about the newborn with a type of ichthyosis.

MAIN INHERITED ICHTHYOSES

Ichthyosis vulgaris

Ichthyosis vulgaris is the most common ichthyosis and its onset during childhood is distinctive. The condition is transmitted as an autosomal dominant trait. The trunk and extensor surfaces of the limbs are the site of fine, white and branny scales which may have a 'pasted on' appearance. The flexures are characteristically spared. The face scales only during early childhood. Palms and soles have prominent markings.

Histologically, it consists of a dense, moderate hyperkeratosis, the absence

Table 15.1 Main inherited ichthyoses

	Mode of inheritance	Gross features	Pathology and epidermal cell kinetics (ep.c.k.)	Associated features	Prognosis
Ichthyosis vulgaris of childhood	Autosomal dominant	Fine scales on trunk and limbs; flexures spared; palms–soles, prominent markings	Mild hyperkeratosis, decreased or absent stratum granulosum, ep.c.k.: normal	Atopy keratosis pilaris	Improves with age
Congenital* ichthyoses — Nigricans†	X-linked	Dark, prominent scales on neck, trunk, limbs; palms–soles: normal	Ep.c.k.: normal (few mitotic figures)	Corneal opacities	
Lamellar†	Autosomal recessive	Generalized large, coarse scales; palms–soles thickened; erythroderma transient	Moderate or marked hyperkeratosis, focal parakeratosis, increased stratum granulosum, prominent rete ridges or acanthosis; many mitotic figures		Remains same or worsens
Erythroderma†	Autosomal recessive	Erythroderma persistent ectropion, eclabion	Ep.c.k.: rapid		
Harlequin fetus	Autosomal recessive	Most severe			

* Or early infancy.
† At birth collodion membrane occasionally.

Table 15.2 Main inherited ichthyosiform hyperkeratoses

		Mode of inheritance	Gross features	Pathology and epidermal cell kinetics (ep.c.k.)	Associated features	Prognosis
Congenital* epidermolytic hyperkeratoses	Generalized (congenital ichthysiform erythroderma bullous form)	Autosomal dominant	Coarse, verrucous scales prominent in flexures; blisters during early life; palms–soles: normal	Marked hyperkeratosis; irregular, coarse keratohyalin granules; vacuolization of the cells in the upper str. Malpighii	Skeletal deformities mental retardation epilepsy, neural deafness	Improves with age
	Localized (linear epidermal nevus) Systematized (ichthyosis hystrix)	Autosomal dominant	Bilateral hyperkeratosis corresponding to Blaschko's lines	Ep.c.k.: rapid		
	Limited (nevus unius lateris)	Autosomal dominant	Unilateral			

* Or early infancy.

139

Table 15.3   Rare inherited ichthyosiform syndromes

		Mode of inheritance	Gross features	Associated features
Congenital (or early infancy)	Sjögren-Larsson	Autosomal recessive	Lamellar ichthyosis-like	Spastic paralysis, epilepsy, mental retardation retinal degeneration dysplasia of tooth enamel
	Rud's	Autosomal recessive	Generalized branny desquamation	Oligophrenia, epilepsy infantilism
	Conradi's	Autosomal recessive	Transient erythroderma micaceous scaling	Stippling of epiphyses short limbs contractures of large joints ophthalmic defects
	Immunodeficiency with short-limbed dwarfism	Autosomal recessive	Micaceous erythroderma; some free areas	Hypogammaglobulinemia defective antibody and cell-mediated immunity
	Tay's	Autosomal recessive	Transient erythroderma, diffuse branny scales	Defective hair hypogammaglobulinemia mental and growth retardation progeria-like appearance
	Psoriasiform erythroderma	Multi factorial	Micaceous erythroderma; some free areas	Psoriasis in childhood
	Erythrokeratodermiae variabiles:			
	(a) Erythrokeratoderma variabilis	Autosomal dominant	Migratory and persistent hyperkeratotic lesions	
	(b) Netherton's	Autosomal recessive	Migratory and persistent hyperkeratotic lesions	Trichorrhexis invaginata atopy
	(c) Ichthyosis linearis circumflexa	Autosomal recessive	Migratory erythematous scaling lesions	
	(d) Symmetrical progressive erythrokeratodermia	Autosomal dominant	Persistent erythematohyperkeratotic plaques	
Childhood	Refsum's	Autosomal recessive	Intermittent generalized branny scaling	Retinitis pigmentosa progressive polyneuritis elevated serum phytanic acid level

of the granular layer being the mark of this ichthyosis. The epidermal proliferation rate is normal. Follicular hyperkeratosis is sometimes associated, or is the only persistent cutaneous manifestation. Atopic disorders are also common in these children or in their families.

Congenital ichthyoses

Congenital ichthyoses include the nigricans form, the lamellar form, the erythrodermatous form and the harlequin fetus, which differ mainly in severity. The affected newborn is commonly of low weight and erythrodermic and often a parchment-like sheet covers the body. All congenital ichthyoses are inherited as autosomal recessive traits, except for the nigricans form which is X-linked and affects males only.

Histologically, congenital ichthyoses are characterized by a variable degree of dense hyperkeratosis with occasional focal parakeratosis, a normal to thickened granular layer, moderate acanthosis and a mild mononuclear infiltrate in the upper dermis. Increased proliferative activity is also demonstrated by many mitotic figures.

Ichthyosis nigricans

Ichthyosis nigricans, frequently called X-linked or sex-linked ichthyosis, has been distinguished from autosomal dominant ichthyosis by Wells and Kerr[5]. The condition exhibits many characteristic features of the congenital ichthyosis group. Often scaling is seen at birth, some cases having a collodion membrane with no ectropion or eclabion. The onset can take place by three months of age, the most extensive involvement of body surface being found in subjects aged more than 20 years. The neck, trunk and lower limbs are invariably affected; also the flexural surfaces often exhibit large scales greater than 4 mm in diameter, and ranging in colour from gray to dark brown. Palms, soles and nails have no relevant abnormalities. In the corneas of preadolescent males small comma- or dot-shaped opacities on the posterior capsule or on the Descemet's membrane, are occasionally detectable[6]. These cause no visual impairment.

Histopathologically there is hyperkeratosis, a prominent granular layer and rete ridges. It resembles the picture observed in lamellar ichthyosis, but with few mitoses. In our opinion, the clinical and histologic appearances of sex-linked ichthyosis, as well as its natural history, are poorly differentiated from those found in autosomal recessive lamellar ichthyosis. In fact, the only differences are that, in the sex-linked type, the palms, soles and epidermal proliferation rates are normal. In practice, however, female patients may be encountered exhibiting the clinical features of ichthyosis nigricans.

On the contrary, the X-linked form is clearly distinguishable from ichthyosis vulgaris because it is recessive, it starts earlier, may exhibit a collodion membrane and worsens with age.

Lamellar ichthyosis

Lamellar ichthyosis is the least severe congenital form. Its enveloping horny layer is thin, collodion-like, and its detachment affects the entire skin, including the flexural surfaces which appear red and scaling; however, the erythroderma gradually subsides within a few months[7]. Large thin scales over the entire body may develop again during subsequent months or years. Palms and soles are thickened.

Erythrodermatous ichthyosis

The erythrodermatous form is a more severe entity than the lamellar one, and it is distinguishable by a dry, scaly mantle with ectropion and eclabion, giving rise to feeding problems. There never are bullae. A generalized erythroderma persists through childhood and beyond, but may become less marked with age.

Harlequin fetus

Harlequin fetus represents the most severe degree of this condition, death occurring *in utero* or shortly after birth. The whole skin is thickened, hyperkeratotic and deeply fissured. The facial features are distorted and the extremities flexed because of extreme cutaneous inelasticity.

Collodion Babies

At birth, children with nigricans, lamellar and erythrodermatous ichthyoses may occasionally be enveloped by a *collodion membrane* (so-called '*collodion babies*')[8]. A collodion baby may be the phenotypic expression of any of the three genotypes mentioned above. These collodion babies show either a gradual transition to nigricans X-linked ichthyosis (in which case they may have the characteristic corneal opacities), or to the lamellar form, or to the erythrodermatous form (if ectropion and eclabion are present). After shedding the membrane, some collodion babies may exhibit a normal skin and consequently some authors believe that the membrane is a persistent periderm coming off at a late stage[9]. However, the histological picture is the same in all cases, there is hyperkeratosis and no retention of nuclei, as in the periderm.

MAIN INHERITED ICHTHYOSIFORM HYPERKERATOSES

Congenital epidermolytic hyperkeratoses

Congenital epidermolytic hyperkeratosis, also called dominant congenital ichthyosiform erythroderma, is an epidermal and dermal dysplasia rather than an ichthyotic disorder. The dermal participation in this disorder is demonstrated by the fact that in localized forms the process recurs, unless the whole skin is removed.

A generalized bullous form and localized forms without blisters exist, but they are essentially the same disorder. The different types possess the same epidermal abnormality histologically and can alternate in succeeding generations.

Generalized form

At the time of birth, the generalized bullous form shows erythroderma and large flaccid bullae or moist raw areas. Later, the skin presents thick gray-brown, often verrucous scales over most of the body, and prominent furrowed hyperkeratosis in the flexural surfaces of the extremities. Vesicles and bullae usually appear during the first years of life. Histologic sections show an abnormal proliferative hyperkeratosis, a characteristic vacuolar degeneration in the middle and upper stratum spinosum and a markedly thickened granular layer, containing a dense collection of irregularly shaped keratohyalin granules. The bulla can be due to separating subcorneally.

Localized form

In localized forms, the papillomatous hyperkeratotic lesions are linear processes or stripes involving one or both sides of the body, with a symmetrical distribution corresponding to Blaschko's lines[10].

Localized systematized form — The systematized form with extensive symmetrical lesions, commonly designated as ichthyosis hystrix[11], is frequently associated with skeletal deformities and central nervous defects such as mental retardation, epilepsy and neural deafness[12].

Localized limited form — In the limited form, linear hyperkeratoses of variable breadth are distributed on the entire upper limbs, most of the trunk and/or the lower limbs, but always on one side only[13].

RARE INHERITED ICHTHYOSIFORM SYNDROMES

There are a number of rare inherited ichthyoses characterized by cutaneous manifestations either alone, such as the group of erythrokeratodermiae variabiles, or in association with other abnormalities. Most of these syndromes are variants of the lamellar or erythrodermic ichthyosis.

143

Congenital syndromes

Sjögren–Larsson syndrome

The Sjögren–Larsson syndrome is an autosomal recessive disorder consisting of congenital lamellar-like ichthyosis. Palms and soles may be thickened. Spastic paralysis occurs during infancy, followed by mental retardation, epilepsy, retinal degeneration and dysplasia of tooth enamel. The histologic features include para- or orthohyperkeratosis, acanthosis and normal or diminished granular layer. The epidermal proliferation rate is increased.

Rud's syndrome

Rud's syndrome is a mild or severe, branny scaling congenital ichthyosis, associated with oligophrenia, epilepsy and infantilism.

Conradi's syndrome

In early infancy, patients with Conradi's syndrome exhibit an erythroderma covered with micaceous scales in a whorl and swirl pattern[3–14]. The condition improves during the first year of life, and sometimes a follicular athrophoderma follows. 'Stippling' of epiphyses, contractures of large joints, short limbs, ophthalmic defects and early death are the other clinical features.

Immunodeficiency with short-limbed dwarfism

Immunodeficiency with short-limbed dwarfism is an autosomal recessive disorder[15–16]. Antibody and cell-mediated immunity is defective. From the first few weeks after birth, there is a severe scaling erythroderma with large coarse scales (Figure 15.1); some areas are free, in others the symptoms rapidly subside for short periods of time then reappear. Histologically the stratum corneum shows parakeratosis and hyperkeratosis and contains some neutrophils. There is an absence of the granular layer, papillomatosis and a moderate acanthosis with many mitoses. There is a mononuclear infiltrate in the upper and papillary dermis.

Tay's syndrome

Tay's syndrome is an autosomal recessive disorder characterized by congenital ichthyosiform erythroderma, pili torti and trichorrhexis nodosa, mental and growth retardation. After some months the erythroderma subsides and the hyperkeratotic scaling is confined to the face, trunk and extensor aspects of the limbs. The palms and soles are thickened. The child shows a progeria-like appearance.

Histologically there is hyperkeratosis with scattered parakeratosis, moderate acanthosis and decreased granular layer. A perivascular lymphocytic infiltrate is observed in the dermis.

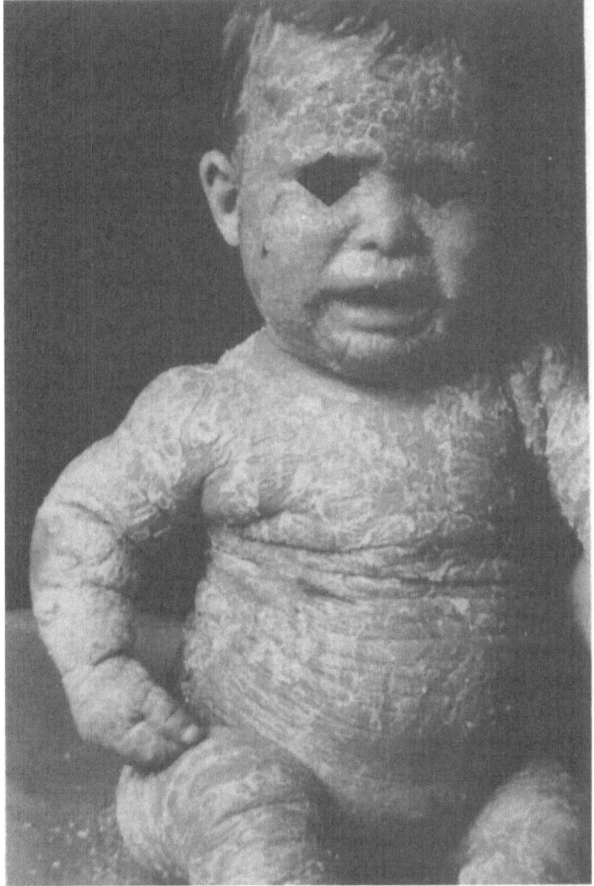

Figure 15.1   Ichthyosiform erythroderma and immunodeficiency with short-limbed dwarfism in a 16-month-old girl

Psoriasiform erythroderma

Psoriasiform erythroderma is really a congenital psoriasis[18], but the gross and histologic features resemble a severe ichthyosiform erythroderma, marked by conspicuous loss of large, micaceous scales for several months. Some normal skin areas are often distinctive. Only the appearance of typical psoriatic patches or pustular psoriasis[19] during childhood permits this diagnosis to be confirmed, as we have also personally observed in our patients.

Erythrokeratodermiae variabiles

Erythrodermia variabilis of Mendes da Costa, Netherton's disease, ichthyosis linearis circumflexa of Comel and symmetrical progressive erythrokeratodermia are rare genodermatoses characterized by redness and figurate or gyrate hyperkeratotic lesions, which change their configuration within days, or within years. All these forms are congenital or appear in early infancy; their course is chronic but improves with age. Probably, these syndromes are variants of lamellar ichthyosis and they all could be included under the descriptive denomination of Erythrokeratodermiae variabiles. In fact, they could be manifestations of the same entity. Their mode of inheritance is still uncertain because the cases reported are too few to allow any definition of the inheritance trait.

Erythrokeratodermia variabilis of Mendes da Costa is an autosomal dominant inherited dermatosis which affects both sexes. It starts at birth or in early infancy with moderate erythrodermic areas changing in size and location from day to day, and rapidly scaling lamellae particularly at the borders; later on, fixed configurate hyperkeratotic plaques arise as such on normal skin. The face, anterior aspect of the body, buttocks and limbs are the commonest sites. The palms and soles may be thickened. Histologic sections show hyperkeratosis with focal parakeratosis, normal granular layer, moderate papillomatosis and acanthosis and a mild perivascular mononucleated infiltrate in the upper dermis. The rate of proliferation is normal[20]. The condition improves with age.

Netherton's syndrome is an inherited, autosomal recessive condition, but almost only females are affected[21,22]. It starts as a transient erythroderma and subsequently develops migratory and fixed cutaneous lesions (similar to those of Erythrokeratodermia variabilis), a characteristic trichorrhexis invaginata on the scalp, eyebrows and eyelashes, and atopy. Palms, soles and nails are normal. The ingestion of nuts causes the exudation of skin lesions. Histologically, hyperkeratosis with parakeratosis, discontinuous stratum granulosum, acanthosis and prominent rete ridges are present. Mononuclear exocytosis and inflammatory infiltrate in the upper dermis are also observed.

Ichthyosis linearis circumflexa of Comel is an autosomal recessive disorder which, from birth or infancy, shows extensive migratory serpiginous and polycyclic lesions of erythema and scaling, with a distinctive double-edged scale at the borders. The course is chronic and the same histopathology is seen as in erythrokeratodermia variabilis.

Symmetrical progressive erythrokeratodermia is an autosomal dominant disorder which starts at birth or during early childhood[23,24]. Erythematohyperkeratotic, sharply outlined areas, occasionally hyperpigmented, usually symmetrical, are present on the extensor surfaces of the limbs (Figure 15.2), buttocks and, occasionally, on the trunk and face. Patches and plaques are persistent and slowly progressive from the beginning. Palms and soles are

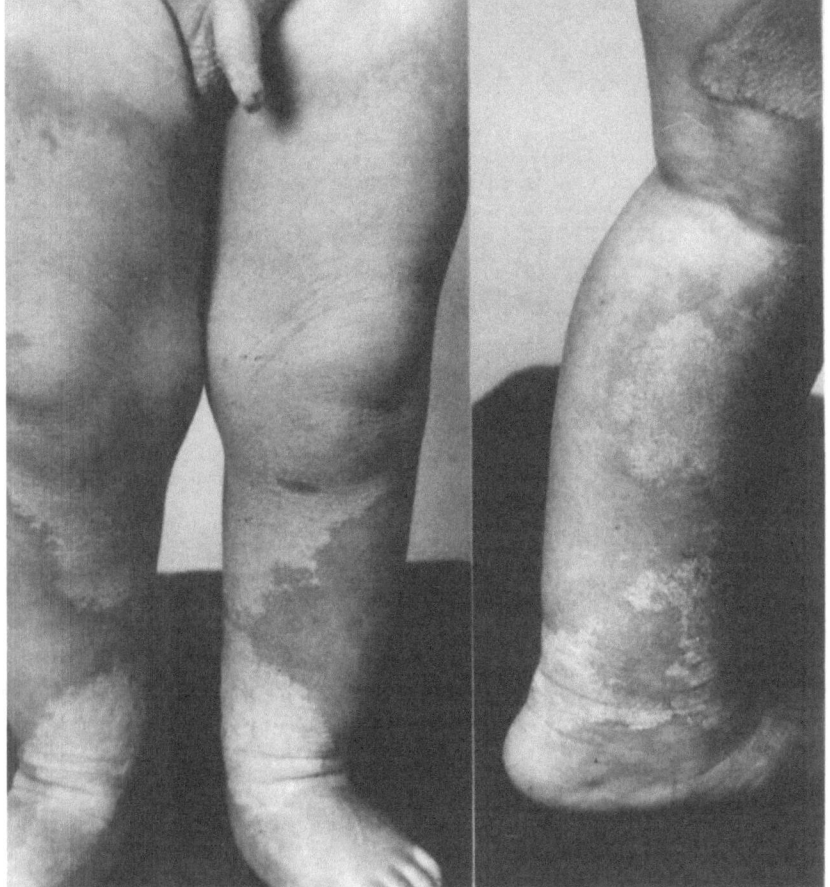

Figure 15.2 Symmetrical progressive erythrokeratodermia started at birth, in a 9-month-old boy

normal. Spontaneous resolution is possible during adulthood. The histopathology is characterized by thick hyperkeratosis, occasionally parakeratosis an increase in the granular layer, and a moderate perivascular infiltrate in the superficial dermis.

Childhood syndromes

Refsum's syndrome

Refsum's syndrome starts in late childhood and beyond. Generalized, branny dirty scales are present in some cases. Retinitis pigmentosa, progressive polyneuritis and cerebellar signs are the cardinal features of this autosomal recessive disorder. Phytanic acid is present in serum and deposits of lipids are found in all tissues.

References

1. Frost, P. and Weinstein, G. D. (1971). Ichthyosiform dermatoses. In T. B. Fitzpatrick, K. A. Arndt, W. H. Clark, A. Z. Eisen, E. J. van Scott and J. H. Vaughan (eds). *Dermatology in General Medicine*, pp. 249–265. (New York: McGraw Hill)

2. Puissant, A. and Beylot, C. (1972). Ichthyoses et états ichtyosiformes. *Encyclopédie Médico-Chirurgicale* (Paris) 12605 A[10], 9

3. Solomon, L. M. and Esterly, N. B. (1973). Scaling disorders. *Neonatal Dermatology*, pp. 110–124. (Philadelphia: W. B. Saunders Co.)

4. Esterly, N. B. (1974). The ichthyoses. In D. J. Demis, R. G. Crounse, R. L. Dobson and J. McGuire. *Clinical Dermatology*, Vol. I, Unit 1-20 to 1-30 (Hargerstown, Mar.: Harper & Row)

5. Wells, R. S. and Kerr, C. B. (1966). Clinical features of autosomal dominant and sex-linked ichthyosis in an English population. *Br. Med. J.*, **1**, 947

6. Jay, B., Blach, R. K. and Wells, R. S. (1968). Ocular manifestations of ichthyosis. *Br. J. Ophthal.*, **52**, 217

7. Bloom, D. and Goodfried, M. S. (1962). Lamellar ichthyosis of the newborn. *Arch. Dermatol.*, **86**, 336

8. Scott, O. L. S. and Stone, D. G. H. (1955). Lamellar desquamation of the new-born ('collodion baby'). *Br. J. Dermatol.*, **67**, 189

9. Reed, W. B., Herwick, R. P., Hasville, D., Porter, P. S. and Conant, M. (1972). Lamellar exfoliation of the newborn. *Arch. Dermatol.*, **105**, 394

10. Jackson, R. (1976). The lines of Blaschko: a review and reconsideration. *Br. J. Dermatol.*, **95**, 349

11. Zeligman, I. and Pomeranz, J. (1965). Variations of congenital ichthyosiform erythroderma. *Arch. Dermatol.*, **91**, 120

12. Solomon, L. M., Fretzin, D. F. and DeWald, R. L. (1968). The epidermal nevus syndrome. *Arch. Dermatol.*, **97**, 273

13. Degos, R., Civatte, J., Belaïch, S. and Tsoïtis (1969). Image histologique particulière de certains naevi verruqueux systématisés. *Ann. Dermatol. Syph.*, Paris, **96**, 361

14. Bodian, E. L. (1966). Skin manifestations of Conradi's disease. *Arch. Dermatol.*, **94**, 743

15. Ammann, A. J. and Hong, R. (1973). Immunodeficiency with short-limbed dwarfism. In E. Stiehm and V. A. Fulginiti (eds.). *Immunologic Disorders in Infants and Children*, p. 261. (Philadelphia: W. B. Saunders Co.)

16. Gatti, R. A., Platt, N., Pomerance, H. H., Hong, R., Langer, L. O., Kay, H. E. M. and Good, R. A. (1969). Hereditary lymphopenic agammaglobulinemia associated with a distinctive form of short-limbed dwarfism and ectodermal dysplasia. *J. Pediat.*, **75**, 675

17. Tay, C. H. (1971). Ichthyosiform erythroderma, hair shaft abnormalities and mental and growth retardation. *Arch. Dermatol.*, **104**, 4

18. Lerner, M. R. and Lerner, A. B. (1972). Congenital Psoriasis. *Arch. Dermatol.*, **105**, 598

19. Henrichsen, L. and Zachariae, H. (1972). Pustular psoriasis and arthritis in congenital psoriasiform erythroderma. *Dermatologica*, **144**, 12

20. Schellander, F. and Fritsch, P. (1969). Variable Erythrokeratodermien. *Arch. Klin. Exp. Dermatol.*, **235**, 241

21. Netherton, E. W. (1958). A unique case of trichorrhexis nodosa-bamboo hairs. *Arch. Dermatol.*, **78**, 483

22. Gianotti, F. (1969). *La maladie de Netherton*. Étude de deux cas et des rapports avec les génodermatoses erythématodesquamatives circinées variables. *Ann. Dermatol.*, **96**, 147

23. Darier, J. (1911). Erythrodermie verruqueuse en nappe, symétrique et progressive. *Bull. Soc. Franç. Dermatol. Syph.*, **22**, 252

24. Hudelo, L., Boulanger-Pilet and Caillau. (1922). Erythrokératodermie verruqueuse en nappes, symétrique et progressive, congénitale. *Bull. Soc. Franç. Dermatol. Syph.*, **29**, 45

16
Follicular Ichthyosiform Disorder

E. WADDINGTON and R. MARKS

INTRODUCTION

Not infrequently clinicians are confronted with patients whose diseases defy diagnosis and which persist largely unchanged for long periods. Even more frustrating is the total inability to make any therapeutic headway in this kind of patient. Disorders of keratinization sometimes qualify for inclusion in this category and we wish to describe such a patient. In so doing we will describe our attempts to understand the tissue basis for his disorder.

THE PATIENT

He was first seen at Cardiff by one of us (Dr. E. Waddington) in 1956. His skin had been dry since the age of 18 months. His father had keratosis pilaris; there was no other relevant family history. Examination at the age of 2 years revealed a normally developed child with generalized follicular horny prominences. The lesions were most pronounced on the cheeks, ears, neck, upper trunk and limbs. All the flexures were involved. There was thickening of the palms and soles.

In 1959 at the age of 5 years he developed milia and pustules on the cheeks. During the next 10 years he had recurrent abscesses and cysts on the neck and upper thighs which produced severe scarring. In contrast the facial lesions did not produce atrophic scars or loss of hair. In 1963 the axillary skin became rugose with increased markings resembling acanthosis nigricans. This has diminished since he developed axillary hair. Many horny plugs were elongated to produce close set filiform spines as in keratosis spinulosa. A biopsy at this

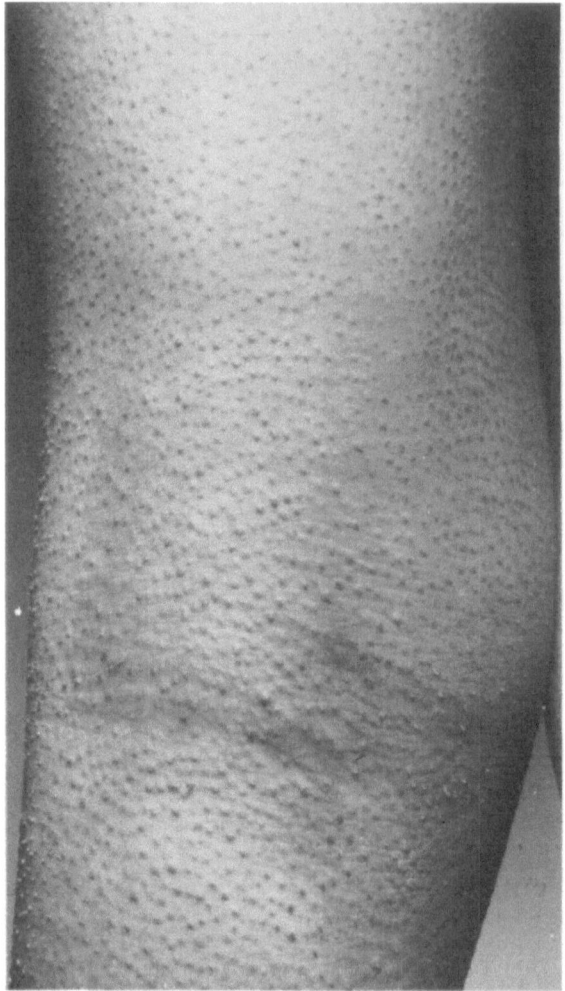

Figure 16.1   Back of knee showing many prominent follicular orifices filled with horny spines

time (aged 9 years) showed follicular and interfollicular hyperkeratosis and some epidermal thickening.

There has been little change during the last 14 years (Figures 16.1–5). Some improvement occurs in warm weather and temporary improvement follows treatment with keratolytics and moisturizers. Vitamin A (systemic and topical) has had no effect. In 1976 he was admitted for further investigations. There was no radiological evidence of bone dysplasia. The serum proteins were normal. The serum triglycerides and cholesterol were normal on three occasions. There was no evidence of essential fatty acid deficiency. Amino acid

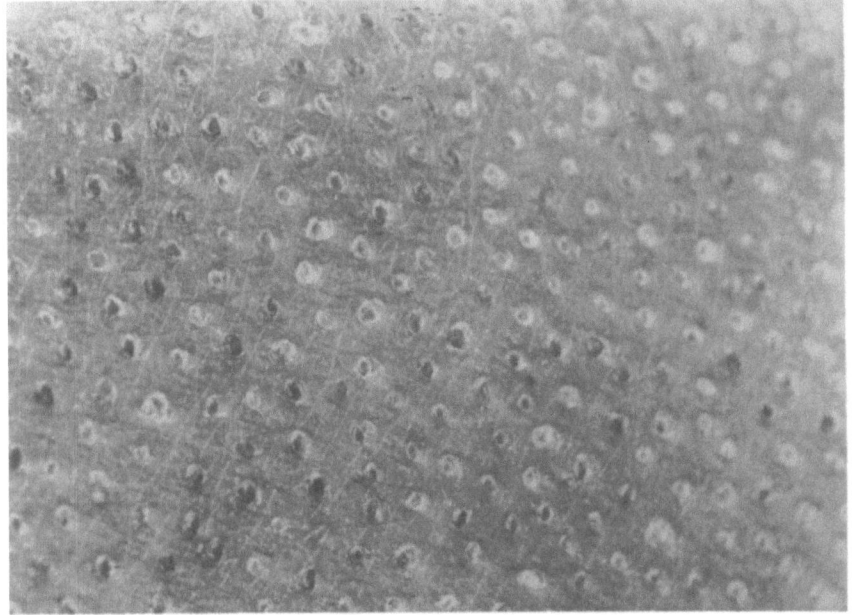

Figure 16.2   Close-up area of thigh to show horny plugs

chromatography of the urine showed no significant abnormality. A skin biopsy showed similar changes to those seen at the age of 9 years (see later).

METHODS AND RESULTS OF INVESTIGATIONS

The following investigations were performed on this patient:

Skin biopsies

1   Light microscopy of formalin fixed tissue

Two biopsies were performed for evaluation of the light microscope appearance of formalin fixed paraffin wax embedded tissue. They both showed some epidermal thickening and concentric lamellae of stratum corneum within the follicular ostia (Figure 16.6). There were no other changes of note.

2   Enzyme histochemistry

A further skin biopsy was taken and fix-frozen in a hexane at $-70°C$. Cryostat sections were then examined for the following enzyme activities:

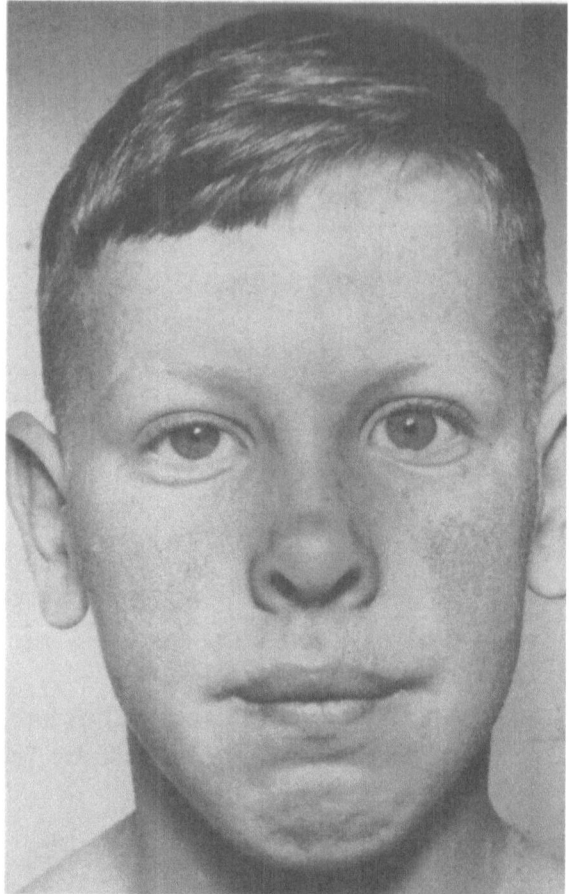

Figure 16.3   Face view to show comedone like plugs over both cheeks

(a) Non-specific esterase
(b) Succinic dehydrogenase
(c) Lactic dehydrogenase
(d) Glucose-6-phosphate dehydrogenase

According to methods outlined
in Chayen *et al.* (1973)[1]

The pattern and intensity of the deposition of reaction products from these reactions did not differ from normal. In particular there did not appear to be any accentuation of enzymic activity associated with keratinization (glucose-6-phosphate dehydrogenase or non-specific esterase) in or near the follicular apparatus.

3   Scanning Electron Microscopy (SEM) of stratum corneum

SEM was performed on both skin surface biopsies obtained using the technique of Marks and Dawber (1971)[2] and on replicas obtained according to the

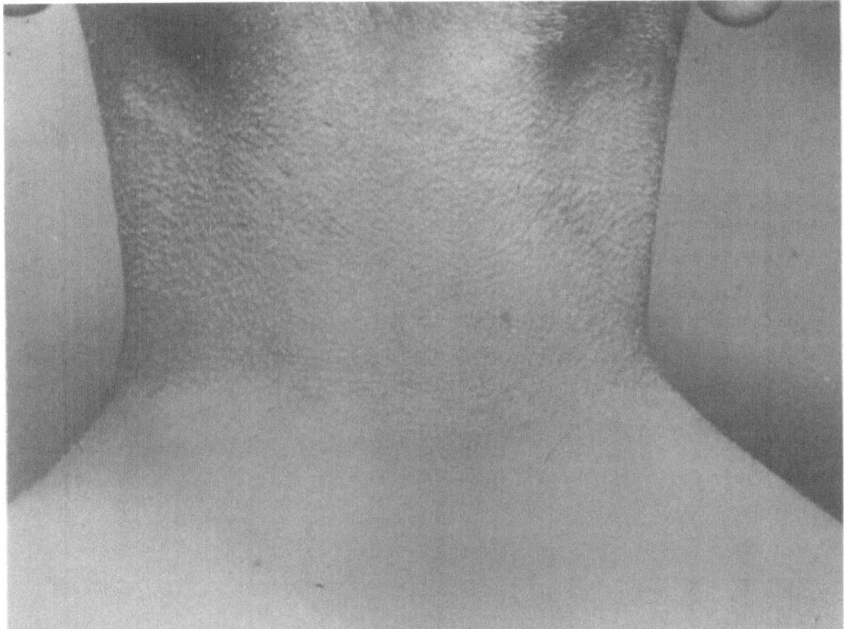

Figure 16.4   Rear view to show the prominent follicular ostia on the back of the neck

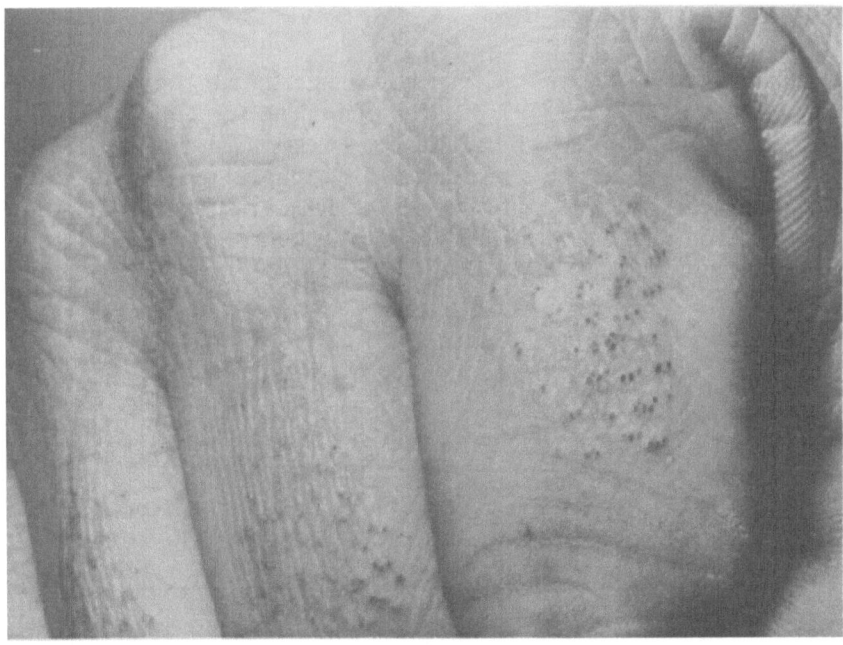

Figure 16.5   Close-up to show comedone like lesions on back of fingers

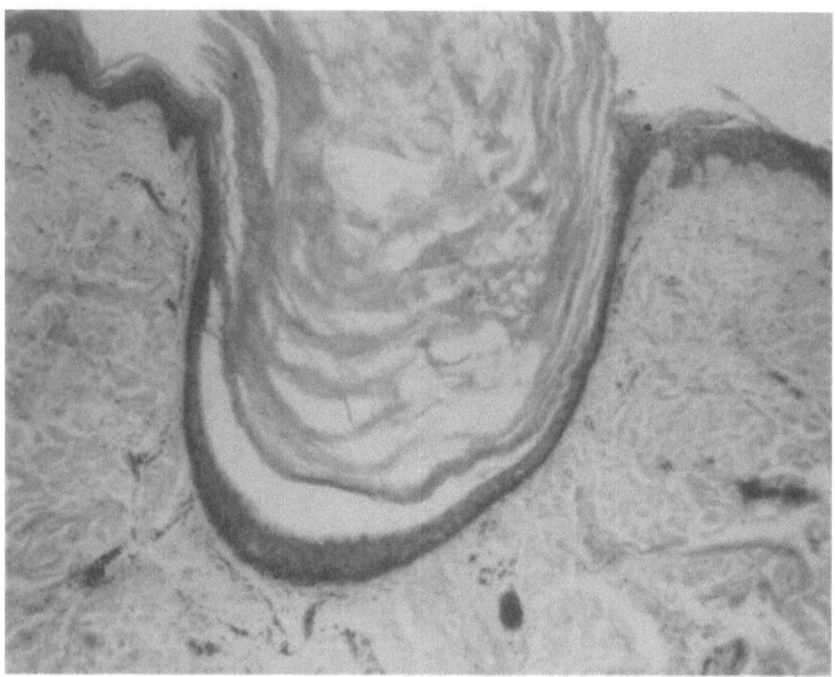

Figure 16.6 Photomicrograph of paraffin section to show widely dilated follicle mouth containing horny plug (*H & E* ×23)

method outlined in Chapter 7. Essentially similar features were noted with both types of specimen. Figures 16.7, 8 and 9 are scanning electron micrographs of skin replicas of this patient. Excellent views were obtained of the follicular corneal plugs which seemed to be penetrated by groups of vellus hairs. The size of the individual follicular orifices was several times greater than normal. The lack of individual corneocyte partial detachment, as normally seen, was quite striking. The surface and shape of the individual corneocyte was quite normal.

4   Rates of precursor incorporation

A keratotome biopsy (0.4 mm thick) was performed on the lateral aspect of the right thigh and the skin sheet was divided into rectangles approximately 70

Table 16.1   **Rates of incorporation of specimens**

Precursor	Result	Normal values ($\pm$ SD)
	(d.p.m./mm²/hr)	
Thymidine	111.0	96 ± 33
Proline	623.3	240 ± 41
Histidine	209.7	107 ± 36

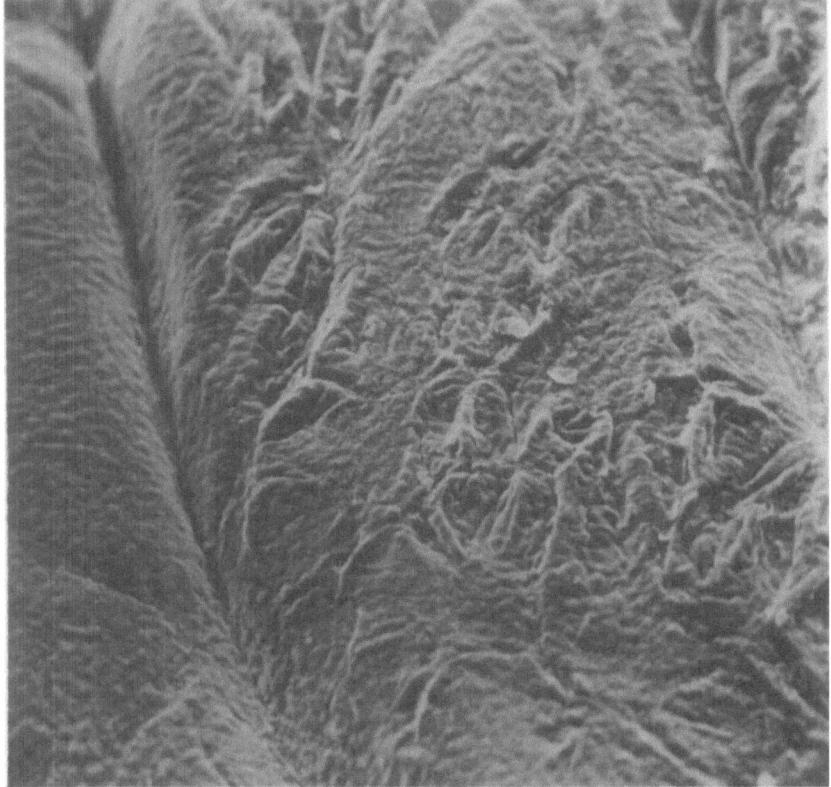

Figure 16.7 Scanning electron micrograph of replica showing surface features of inter-follicular skin. Those scales present are closely adherent and few are in the process of desquamation (×104)

mm². These were incubated *in vitro* for 4 hours in the presence of tritiated thymidine, proline and histidine according to the technique described by Holt and Marks (1976)[3] and also in Chapters 4 and 6 in this symposium. The rates of incorporation and the normal values are given in Table 16.1.

COMMENT

The following clinical diagnoses have been considered: Pityriasis rubra pilaris (PRP); keratosis pilaris; generalized comedone naevus; and ichthyosis with a pronounced follicular component.

The first diagnosis PRP can be excluded both because of the lack of any reddening of the skin, psoriasiform patches or hyperkeratotic change on palms and soles and because of the normal rate of thymidine incorporation indicating a normal rate of epidermal cell production[4]. Keratosis pilaris may be quite

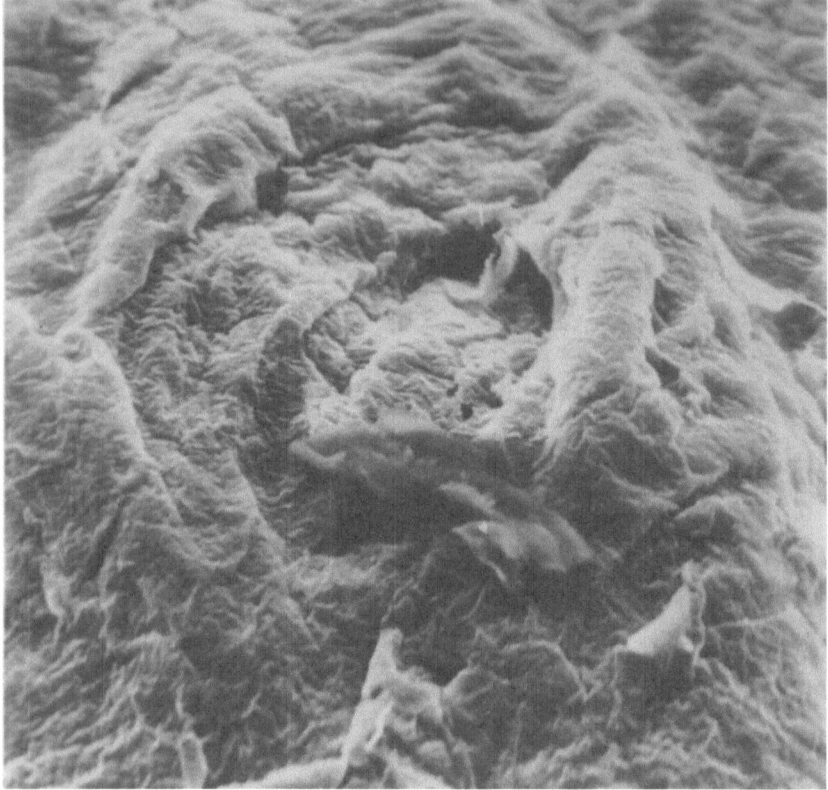

Figure 16.8   Scanning electron micrograph of replica of sweat duct showing closely adherent scale on the surface (×495)

severe but the degree of involvement seen in this patient would be unique for this diagnosis.

In some areas the lesions did in fact resemble comedones (Figures 16.2 and 5) and as can be seen from this patient's history in some areas he did develop inflammatory acne type lesions (as is seen in areas of comedone naevus)[5]. For this reason the diagnosis of generalized comedone naevus has to be seriously considered despite the fact that this young man's condition was so widespread. However, the generalized xeroderma and the apparent deficiency of corneo-cytes caught in the process of desquamation in the scanning electron micrographs of skin surface replicas, suggest to us that this patient is in fact suffering from a type of ichthyosis. Supportive evidence comes from the high rate of proline incorporation seen in the biochemical studies performed. The level of incorporation is 2.5 times normal and for as yet unexplained reasons heightened proline incorporation is seen in many varieties of ichthyotic disorders (see Chapter 4).

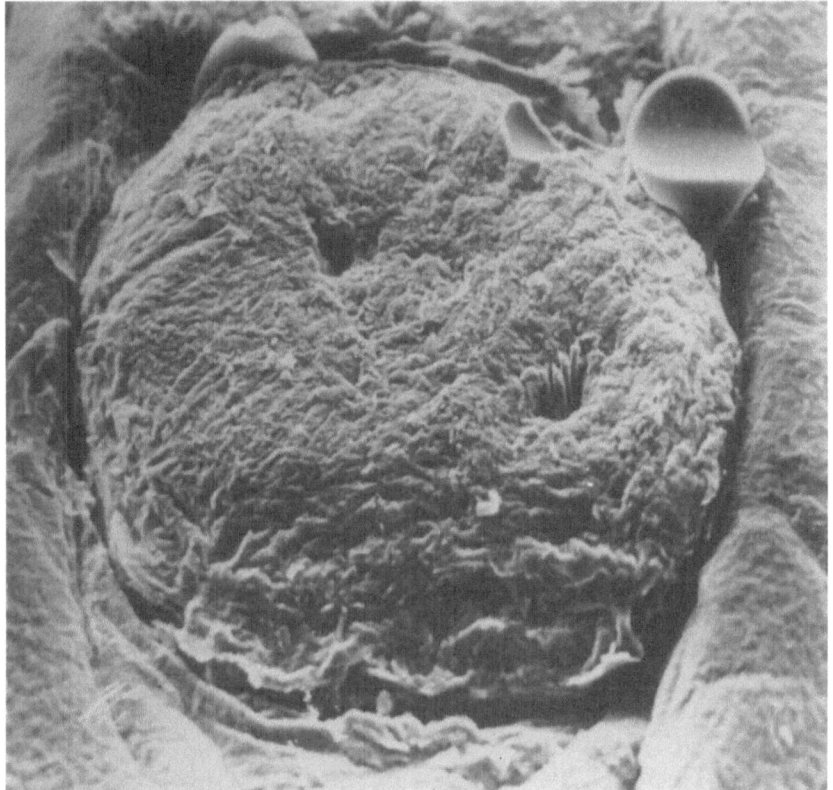

Figure 16.9 Scanning electron micrograph of replica showing a widely dilated follicular ostium penetrated by a cluster of vellus hair (×100)

References

1. Chayen, J., Bitensky, L. and Butcher, R. (1973). *Practical Histochemistry* (London: John Wiley & Sons)
2. Marks, R. and Dawber, R. P. R. (1971). Skin surface biopsy. An improved technique for examination of the stratum corneum. *Br. J. Dermatol.*, **84,** 117
3. Holt, P. J. A. and Marks, R. (1976). Epidermal architecture, growth and metabolism in acromegaly. *Br. Med. J.*, **1,** 496
4. Marks, R. and Griffiths, W. A. D. (1973). The epidermis in pityriasis rubra pilaris: A comparison with psoriasis. *Br. J. Dermatol.*, **89,** Supplement 9, 19
5. Leppard, B. and Marks, R. (1973). Comedone naevus. A report of nine cases. Transactions of St. John's Hospital Dermatological Society, **59,** 45

17
Two Cases of Unusual Ichthyosis

R. HOWELL

INTRODUCTION

Two cases of severe and unusual ichthyosis are described which have been reported previously[1,2]. The present note summarizes the findings.

Case 1   J.H.L., Male, Aged 60

History — In infancy developed blisters on the fingers and toes. In childhood developed hyperkeratotic areas on palms and soles. Blisters and nodules developed on the trunk. Between ages 13–37 he was bedridden in hospital and completely incapacitated. In 1955, he had a coronary thrombosis. In March 1956, excision of hyperkeratotic areas and grafting on palms and soles resulted in ability to lead independent life. In 1975 he died suddenly, probably from coronary thrombosis. There was no relevant family history.

Clinical findings — There was gross hyperkeratosis, with blisters in areas on hands and feet. There was onychia of hands and feet, multiple follicular keratoses, acne, comedones, cystic lesions and lipomata on trunk and limbs. Hyperkeratotic plaques on tongue.

Histology — The lesions were entirely epidermal. Localized epithelial hyperplasia with vacuolation in prickle and granular cells causing sub-corneal bullae.

Comment — Various diagnostic titles have been given. A variant of pachyonychia congenita has been suggested[3].

Case 2   E.J.M., Female, Aged 5

History — The skin was normal at birth. At 10 days, mild peeling of skin occurred. At 3 weeks, there was thickening of skin of face, elbows and knees. Subsequently developed widespread areas of well demarcated hyperkeratosis on face, scalp, trunk and limbs. The palms and soles were not affected. Hair, nails and teeth normal. General health and development normal. There was no relevant family history.

Examination — Large well demarcated areas of hyperkeratotic skin as stated above.

Histology — Regular epidermal hyperplasia and hyperkeratosis.

Comment — The affected areas are fixed, excluding erythroderma variabilis. Two families with a similar type of ichthyosis and affected siblings are known[4].

References

1. Howell, R. (1973a). *Br. J. Dermatol.*, **89,** Supplement 9, 57
2. Howell, R. (1973b). *Br. J. Dermatol.*, **89,** Supplement 9, 62
3. Wells, R. S. (1973). Personal Communication
4. Wells, R. S. (1972). Personal Communication

Section 3
Treatment

18
The Effect of Urea on the Skin with Special Reference to the Treatment of Ichthyosis

G. SWANBECK

INTRODUCTION

Urea is a simple organic compound, the first ever synthesized in a laboratory. It is readily soluble in water. It is a hydrogen bond breaker and has been used extensively in protein chemistry as a denaturing agent. It has also been used as a solvent for epidermal keratin[1]. In 1968 it was shown that urea strongly increased the water-binding capacity of scales from psoriatic patients[2]. Urea is also one of the major constituents of the water-soluble fraction of the normal horny layer[3]. This fraction is supposed to be the moisturizing factor which keeps a certain amount of water bound to the horny layer to make it soft and pliable. This fraction occurs in a much lower concentration in the psoriatic scales and possibly also in the scales of some forms of ichthyosis. On this basis I thought that if it were possible to apply a high concentration of urea in a cream base, it might be a useful therapy in ichthyosis vulgaris. Preliminary clinical trials were made which showed that this was the case[2]. With the

Table 1 Urea treatment of ichthyosis vulgaris in order to obtain the most rapid clinical improvement

1	Bath
2	Dry for 5–15 minutes
3	Apply urea cream in excess without rubbing
4	Wait 10–15 minutes
5	Wipe off excess cream
6	Repeat daily for one week
7	Thereafter apply urea cream daily in sufficient amount

following regimen most patients with even a severe ichthyosis vulgaris will be cleared in about one week (Table 18.1).

Among the controlled double-blind studies on the clinical efficacy mention should be made of two. One is an unpublished study made in Sweden by Flodén and Leczinsky[4], the results of which are illustrated in Figure 18.1. In

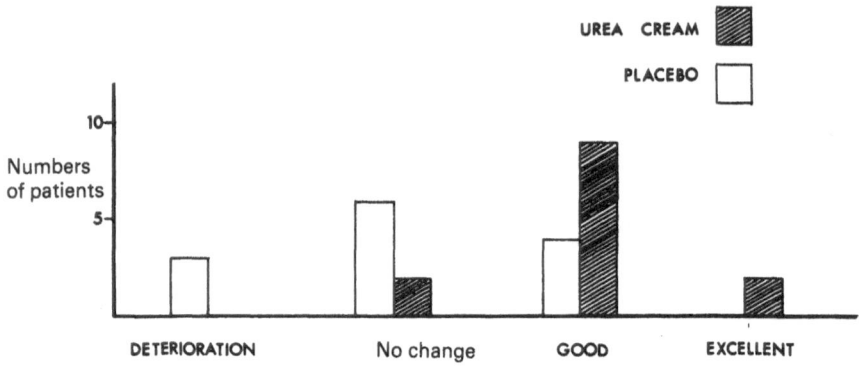

DATA FROM FLODÉN AND LECZINSKY.

Figure 18.1 Double-blind half-side study of the clinical effect of 10% urea cream (Calmurid®) versus vehicle in 13 patients. The physicians evaluation after 3 weeks of treatment is indicated.

another study Pope *et al.* compared a urea cream with three other keratolytic agents. It was shown that used properly urea cream is a very effective agent for treating ichthyosis vulgaris. In an elegant study Grice *et al.*[6] have studied clinical efficacy and effect on transepidermal water loss and water binding capacity of scales removed from patients treated with urea cream. They were able to show that the water binding capacity of the scales several days after the last treatment was considerably higher for urea-treated skin and the transepidermal water loss was reduced.

MATERIALS AND METHODS

In experiments with urea creams I have used two types of additives to improve the property of the cream. One is lactic acid buffered to a pH between 3 and 4. In this way the cream will keep sterile without any other preservative and the skin will probably be more resistant to infections. Lactic acid also has other interesting properties in respect to ichthyosis[7]. Another additive which is of some interest is sodium chloride. Sodium chloride has in itself the ability to increase the water-binding capacity of the horny layer. If we combine sodium chloride and urea the water-binding capacity increases significantly. About equal concentration by weight of urea and sodium chloride gives a water-binding capacity that is far higher than for any of the compounds alone at a

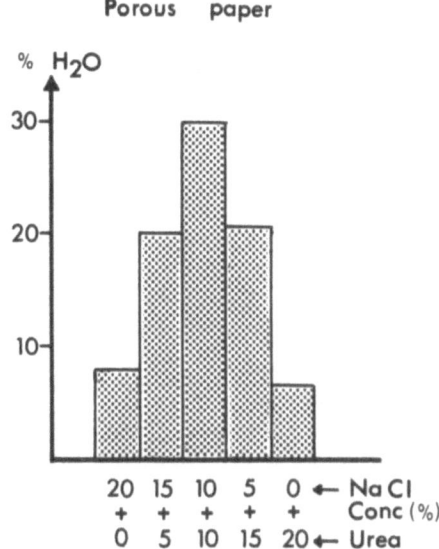

Figure 18.2 Water uptake of porous paper immersed in different solutions of NaCl and urea, dried overnight and equilibrated for 48 hours in a relative humidity of 75%. Similar results are obtained if psoriatic or ichthyotic scales are used instead of porous paper

comparable concentration (Figure 18.2). Evidently there is some synergistic effect between sodium chloride and urea with regard to water binding. With the combination of sodium chloride and urea in concentrations of about 10% of each, a very high degree of moisturizing effect can be obtained. In our clinical experiments we have tried urea creams on congenital ichthyosiform erythroderma but only a minor improvement has been obtained.

COMMENT

It is tempting to speculate that in ichthyosis vulgaris the defect of the epidermis is such that when the body is in the amnion fluid the skin functions properly and the child is born with a normal looking skin. After the child has been washed several times by the mother and been in the dry atmosphere of the normal milieu, the horny layer starts becoming dry, does not desquamate and scales are built up. By restoring the water-binding capacity of the horny layer by adding low molecular weight compounds like urea and lactic acid the defect is partly compensated for and the skin starts functioning more normally and desquamates more easily.

One effect of applying high concentrations of urea to the skin regularly is a certain decrease in cell renewal in the epidermis[8]. However, by using a 10% urea cream Wohlrab only found a decrease of about 10% in cell renewal[9].

Whether this is due to the hydrating properties of urea or some effect on cell metabolism is not known. It should, however, be pointed out that an occlusive dressing alone decreases the cellular renewal in epidermis[10].

References

1. Rudall, K. M. (1952). The proteins of the mammalian epidermis. *Adv. Protein Chem.*, **7**, 253
2. Swanbeck, G. (1956). A new treatment of ichthyosis and other hyperkeratotic conditions. *Acta Dermatol. (Stockholm)*, **48**, 123
3. Spier, H. W. and Pascher, G. (1955). Die Wasserlöslichen Bestandteile der peripheren Hornschicht. Quantitative Analysen. I. Allgemeine stickstoffhaltige Substanzen. *Arch. Dermatol. Syph.*, **199**, 411
4. Flodén, C. H. and Leczinsky, C.-G. (1969). Pharmacia Research Report L 23565
5. Pope, F. M., Rees, J. K., Wells, R. S. and Lewis, K. G. S. (1972). Out-patient treatment of ichthyosis, a double-blind trial of ointments. *Br. J. Dermatol.*, **86**, 291
6. Grice, K., Sattar, H. and Baker, H. (1973). Urea and retionic acid in ichthyosis and their effect on transepidermal water loss and water holding capacity of stratum corneum. *Acta Dermat. (Stockholm)*, **53**, 114
7. Van Scott, E. J. and Yu, R. J. (1974). Control of keratinization with α-hydroxy acids and related compounds. I. Topical treatment of ichthyotic disorders. *Arch. Dermatol.*, **110**, 586
8. Wohlrab, W. and Schiemann, S. (1976). Untersuchungen zum Mechanismus der Harnstoffwirkung auf die Haut. *Arch. Dermatol. Res.*, **255**, 23
9. Wohlrab, W. (1976). Personal communication
10. Baxter, D. L. and Stoughton, R. B. (1970). Mitotic index of psoriatic lesions treated with anthralin, glucocorticosteroid and occlusion only. *J. Invest. Dermatol.*, **54**, 410

19
Pharmaceutical Developments in the Production of Delivery Systems for Treating Ichthyotic Conditions

P. J. W. AYRES

HISTORICAL BACKGROUND

Urea is thought to be responsible for the changes in histological appearance and permeability of mammalian skin described in this study. This relatively simple molecule was first found in urine in 1773 and synthetically prepared from cyanic acid and ammonia by Wohler in 1828.

It is impossible to establish who first used this compound in the treatment of pathological conditions of the skin since it is shrouded in folklore and lay medicine. Certainly the use of 'aged urine' (concentrated by evaporation), was popular for the treatment of warts, bunions, chilblains, brittle nails and scaling of the skin and extended well into the middle 30's of this century. This lay treatment seems explicable on the basis of present day knowledge of the fundamental effects of urea on the keratinized cell layer of mammalian skin.

The use of urea as a bactericide for wounds was recommended by Symmers and Kirk in 1915[1] and later by Robinson in 1936[2]. Rattner reported on the use of urea in a hand cream in 1943[3]. More recently Swanbeck[4] has used a 10% urea cream for the treatment of ichthyosis and other conditions. Stewart et al.[5] investigated the use of 10% urea creams in certain stubborn dermatoses with favourable results.

The fundamental mechanisms involved when urea is applied to the skin must lie within the disciplines of physics. However, it is reasonable to divide the effects at the levels where inter-molecular structural changes take place and

167

those where their interacting forces bring about changes in molecular configurations and hence changes in the physical properties of molecules. At present there is insufficient evidence available to suggest that biochemical interactions play a significant role in the observed effects of urea on the skin. Unfortunately, some physical properties common to a very large number of chemical compounds are often described as though unique to a single one. Hence the primary effect is often listed amongst many other properties which in fact are the result of the primary one.

The primary effect of a concentrated aqueous solution of urea on an insoluble protein is due to the very great hydrogen bond forming power of this medium. The intra-chain hydrogen bonds of the polypeptide helix of the proteins will be weakened and the unfolding of this helical structure will result in reduction of the hydrophobic properties of the protein molecules which will pass into aqueous solution. This capacity for breaking such hydrogen bonds within the structure of a protein is a major factor in making urea a powerful denaturating agent for protein. However, it should be borne in mind that denaturation of the protein does not necessarily result as it is possible to dissolve both insulin and ribonuclease in high molarity solutions of urea without destroying the biological activity of either[6]. This physical effect of hyper-molar urea on the protein was observed and has been used in structural investigations on proteins for many years.

The introduction of urea for dermatological use led to some controversy as to whether the long-term application of high concentrations of urea should be recommended. Part of this controversy was based on observations made by the immersion of epidermis in concentrated urea under *in vitro* conditions[7]. The fact that the tissue became gel-like in consistency under the conditions described was hardly very surprising and could in no way be translated to those effects that might take place under *in vivo* topical application.

INTRODUCTION

The purpose of this paper is to describe a topical preparation that has therapeutic properties itself and is also a versatile drug delivery system.

The protein solubilizing properties of urea referred to in the historical background are very useful in a drug delivery system. It is well known that urea has the property of solubilizing hydrophobic compounds. This solubilization effect may be the result of a simple change in the hydrophobic bonding of the compound, or the formation of complexes with urea or due to physical change with the formation of inclusion complexes referred to as clathrates. An example of increased solubilization of a hydrophobic substance is that of Cortisol and Figure 19.1 shows in graphic form the increased solubility of Cortisol with increasing concentrations of aqueous urea. The solubility of Cortisol in water at 20°C is in the order of 0.3 mg per ml, whereas the solubility is increased to 7.0 mg per ml at a concentration of 9.2 molar urea.

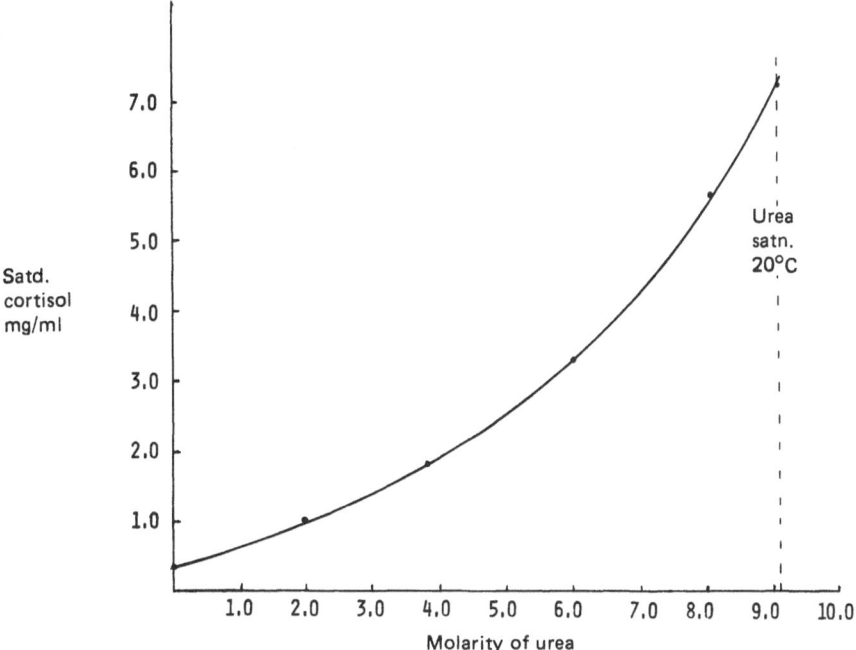

Figure 19.1 Cortisol saturation in aqueous urea at 20 °C

This alteration in the hydrophobic characteristics of a known polar substance such as Cortisol is also extended to other molecules. It was observed that a polysaccharide powder saturated with a lipid shows a linear displacement of the lipid by the addition of water since the polysaccharide has a higher water affinity than it has lipid affinity. However, if a hyper-molar urea solution is used to displace the lipid, a distinct change in the hydrophilic/lipophobic characteristics of the polysaccharide takes place. Figure 19.2 shows the linear displacement of lipid from a saturated polysaccharide particle by water. Displacement continues up to 90% whereas in the case of 9.5 molar urea solution displacement of lipid ceases at approximately 45%. This displacement curve for urea solution is quoted here in millilitres of water corrected for the volume occupied by urea. It can, therefore, be seen that the effect of urea on the polysaccharide particle is virtually to form an ambiphilic particle from a solid particulate material.

Urea in solution is a mono-acidic base and an aqueous solution tends to hydrolyse into carbon dioxide and ammonia. This characteristic of decomposition which, of course, is temperature dependent, limits the applicability of a urea solution in a topical preparation that has to be stored with a reasonable shelf life. As would be expected the acidification of an aqueous urea solution accelerates this decomposition and Figure 19.3 shows the ammonia production by hyper-molar urea solutions buffered at different pH's and stored at

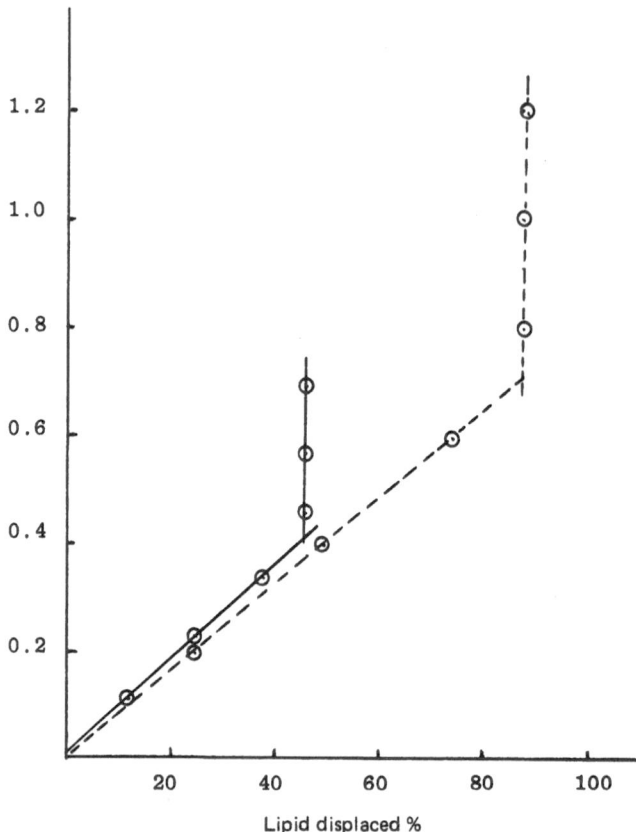

Figure 19.2 Displacement of Lipid from a polysaccharide. By water ○————○, by 9.5M urea ○————○

30°C for varying periods of time. Clearly the slope of decomposition is reduced as the pH is raised. The stability of hyper-molar urea solution is considerably increased by absorbing the solution into a polysaccharide particle. This particle can then be suspended in a continuous lipid phase with the correct incorporation of surfactants with a hydrophile/lipophile balance value suitable to maintain an aqueous–in lipid, continuous phase. The result of this is a compartmentalized system where the urea is in a more stabilized state and the polysaccharide has been altered in its hydrophobic/lipophilic properties to become what might be termed an ambiphilic matrix.

In order to extrapolate the *in vitro* observation that urea will form an ambiphilic particle with a polysaccharide to that of compounds encountered in an *in vivo* environment, two topical preparations containing 10% and 20% urea were applied to the dorsal and ventral skin areas of the forearms in a number of human volunteer subjects. A weighed quantity of preparation was applied to the skin using an impervious finger stall and the material was rubbed

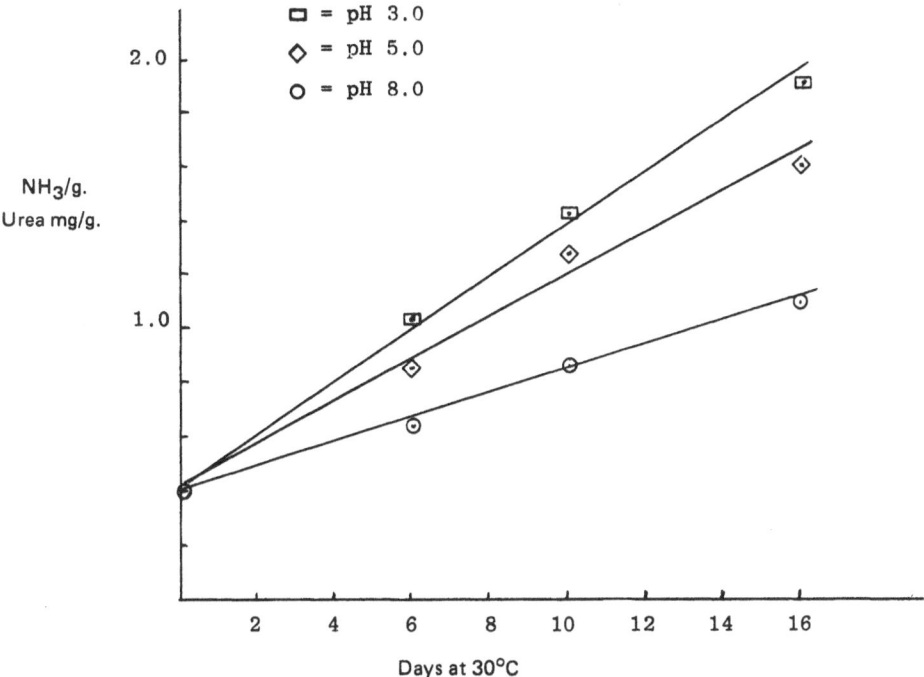

Figure 19.3   Ammonia production in solution at 30°C

into a defined area for a fixed period of time. The excess preparation was removed with a spatula and the non-absorbed material weighed. Figure 19.4 shows the mean and standard deviation of the results obtained. It can be seen that there is a clear increase in total cream uptake by the skin with an increasing concentration of urea compared to that obtained with a soft white paraffin as a value of 1.

This simply derived data as given here indicated that further, more controlled experiments should be carried out. The following describes some *in vivo* experiments on young piglets using a topical preparation containing 10% urea, compared with that of two other preparations, one using propylene glycol as a penetrant in a lipid emulsion (FAPG) and that of a plain aqueous lipid cream.

EXPERIMENT AND RESULTS

Five-week-old piglets were shaved and acclimatized over a period of a week to get them used to wearing a simple wide mesh gauze covering over their back skin where the cream preparations were to be applied. The dorsal skin was washed and marked out into 3 × 3 cm zones on each side of the mid-line.

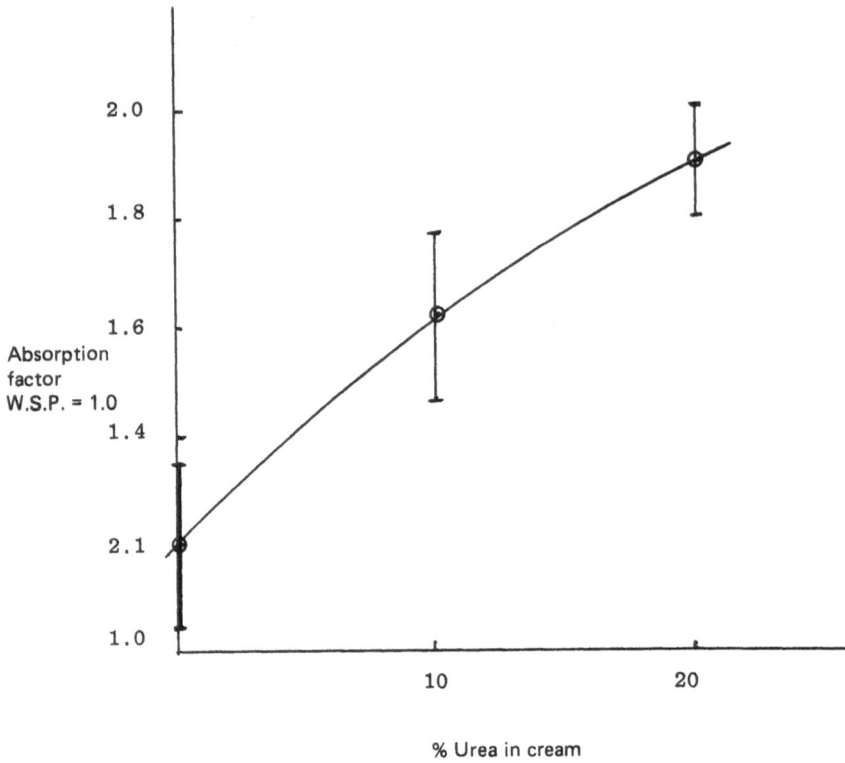

Figure 19.4 Cream absorption *in vivo* by human skin in the presence of urea

0.5 g samples of the creams were applied and rubbed into the skin surface by means of a finger protected by an impervious stall. The creams were applied twice daily with an interval of 8 hours between. After 4 days of application the animals were sacrificed and skin sections from the various areas removed for histological examination. Standard paraffin blocks were prepared for haematoxylin and eosin staining and cryostat sections were cut for sudan-red lipid staining.

Figures 19.5, 6, and 7 show skin sections stained with haematoxylin and eosin at a magnification of ×565. As can be seen in Figure 19.7 compared with Figures 19.5 and 19.6 the effect of a 10% urea preparation is to cause a clear swelling and increased depth of epidermal ridges. In addition there is the appearance of vacuoles where defatting of the section has removed lipid deposits within the epidermis.

Some vacuoles can be seen to be present in the section where the propylene glycol penetrant was used. However, they are very much fewer in number than those observed for the 10% urea preparation. The epidermal thickness was measured over 1.5 cm length sections of skin at intervals of 20 microns. The measurement of epidermal thickness was divided into two groups to cover the

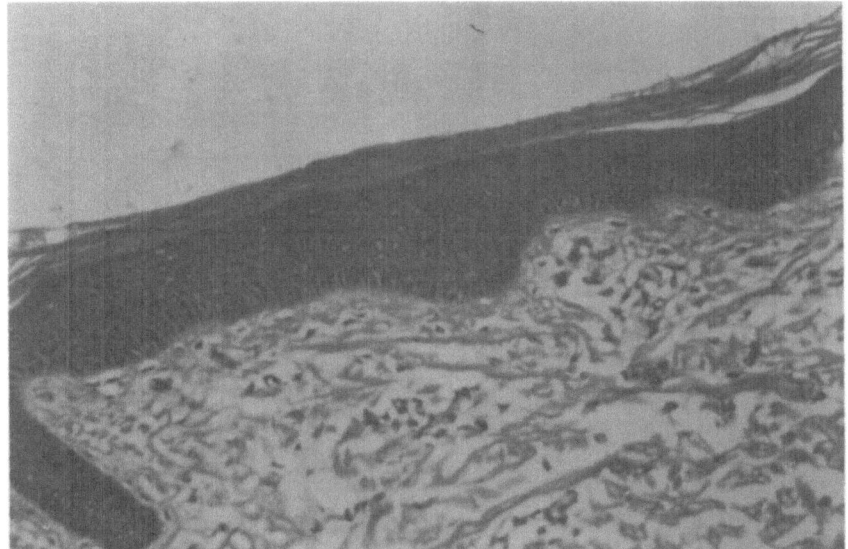

Figure 19.5   Piglet skin section after 4 days application of aqueous/lipid cream. H. & E. stain

thickness of 10–60 microns and 70–180 microns and treated as two total population groups over the 1.5 cm sections and expressed as a percentage of the total length of the section. It can be seen from Table 19.1 that a very clearly defined increase in thickness occurs with the 10% urea preparation compared

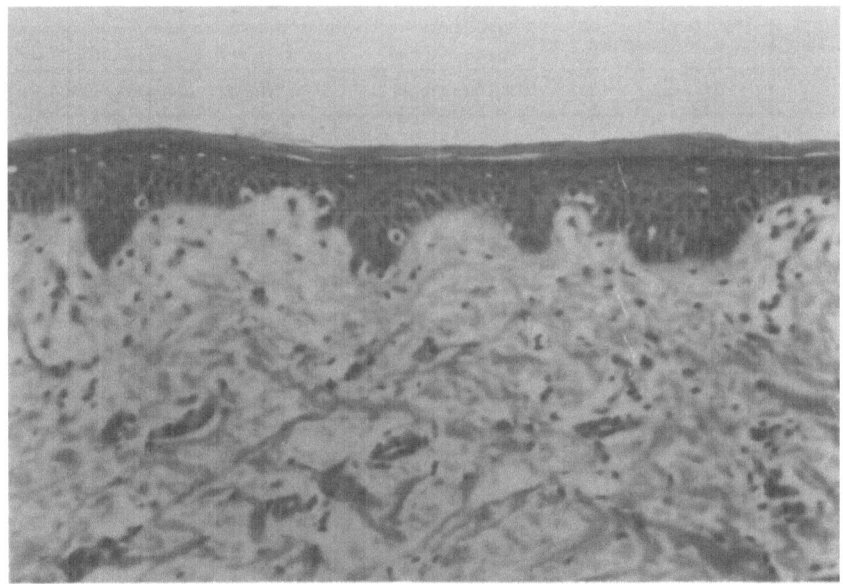

Figure 19.6   Piglet skin section after 4 days application of FAPG/ lipid cream. H. & E. stain

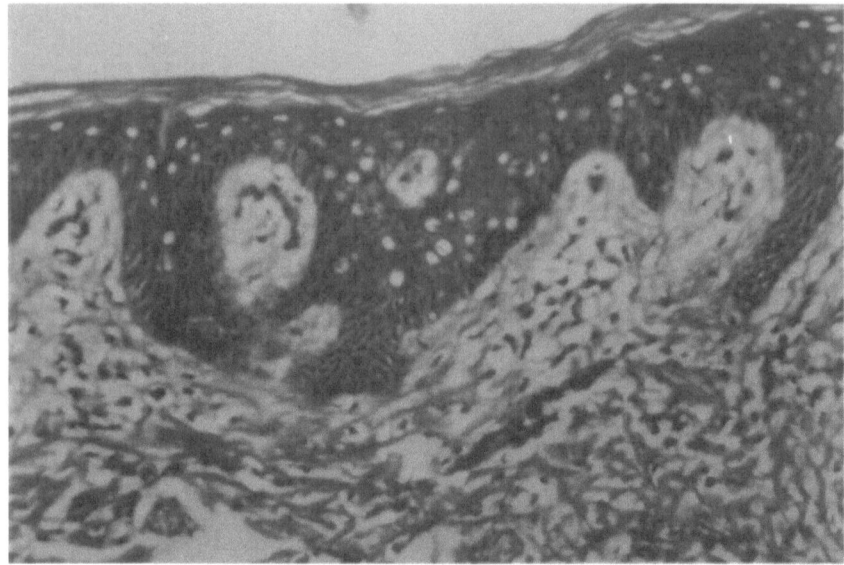

Figure 19.7 Piglet skin section after 4 days application of 10% urea cream. H. & E. stain

to that of a simple aqueous emulsion cream or the preparation containing propylene glycol. Cryostat sections were stained for lipid with sudan red. Vacuoles that were evident in the haematoxylin and eosin sections were heavily stained by the sudan dye in the skin treated with the 10% urea preparation.

Table 19.1 Epidermal thickness

Thickness	10% Urea cream	FAGP/lipid	Aqueous/lipid cream
10–60 micron	47	54	69
70–180 micron	53	46	31

DISCUSSION

The stratum corneum is the limiting membrane that restricts the movement of chemical substances either inward or outward from the epidermis. Once the stratum corneum has been passed the further passage of substances through the epidermis and hence to the dermis and capillaries can take place. When hydrated, the stratum corneum contains approximately 75% water, 20% protein and 5% lipid. If changes in the hydrophobic/lipophilic properties of the stratum corneum are induced then molecular diffusion for polar and non-polar molecules could be quite drastically changed. Their movement would reflect the particular change of the stratum corneum in the direction of increased affinity for water or increased affinity for lipid. Therefore, providing variable dual pathways of aqueous and lipid nature for the transportation of substances with widely different partition coefficients. The histological findings in this investigation indicate that these changes are induced in practice and that not only is the barrier effect of the stratum corneum reduced or overcome, but there is also a lipid depot formation in the epidermis. This provides an important diffusional pathway for drugs that have a partition coefficient in favour of lipid materials.

The changes in the cellular architecture of the epidermis are in keeping with the observations of Montagna[8] who found that 5.0 molar urea causes swelling of the epidermal cells beneath the stratum granulosum and that the stratum corneum was swollen but not disturbed structurally. It is generally agreed that diffusion through this horny layer is a passive process affected mainly by physical factors. Therefore, the topical use of material based on the system described could be of great value as both a drug delivery system and in the treatment of certain disorders, particularly the ichthyoses. Where hyperkeratotic conditions require the delivery of drugs to the epidermis to alter biochemical pathways the former becomes of particular value. In ichthyotic conditions which respond well to hydration the application of this preparation combines the advantage of hydration with the affinity for increased lipid and the occlusive effect of such lipid in maintaining the hydration of the skin.

The induced binding of lipid by increased physical surface forces will have an advantage over that of a simple occlusion by a lipid cream. As referred to earlier, the formation of variable dual pathways of lipid and aqueous nature allows the transportation of substances of widely differing partition coefficients. It is considered that the experimental evidence submitted here confirms the available clinical data in the dermatological field that there are advantages in the use of urea within a compartmentalized system for the treatment of the ichthyoses and other dermatological disorders.

Although a variety of materials have been used as vehicles to accelerate the penetration of topically applied drugs, these substances have a number of disadvantages. Many are volatile and cannot be maintained in adequate concentrations for topical application. Others are irreversible protein denaturants and as such the resultant damage under prolonged use cannot be predicted. It has been shown that 8 molar urea can be more effective as a penetrant than DMSO[9] and in addition the major advantage for urea is that it is not allergenic and at high concentration shows some bacteriostatic activity. In addition urea does not necessarily, when optimum concentrations are used, denature the protein that it comes in contact with. The properties described and its non-toxicity, therefore, make urea the basis of a most acceptable drug delivery system. The advantages of percutaneous delivery over those of systemic administration of substances for dermatological treatment are widely accepted.

This presentation has concentrated on the fundamental processes that occur when a particular urea-containing system is applied to the skin. The physical properties of the material and the experimental evidence that the horny barrier can be overcome make one wonder whether we may shortly be able to deliver therapeutic substances for systemic administration via the skin.

References

1. Symmers, W. St. C. and Kirk, T. S. (1915). Urea as a bactericide in its application in the treatment of wounds. *Lancet*, **2,** 1237
2. Robinson, W. (1936). The use of urea to stimulate healing in chronic purulent wounds. *Am. J. Surg.*, **33,** 192
3. Rattner, H. (1943). The use of urea in hand creams. *Arch. Dermatol. Syph.*, **48,** 47
4. Swanbeck, G. (1968). A new treatment of ichthyosis and other hyperkeratotic conditions. *Acta Dermatol. Vener.*, **48,** 123
5. Stewart, W. D., Danio, J. L. and Maddin, W. S. (1969). Urea cream. *Cutis*, **5** (10), 1241
6. Hvidt, A. and Linderstrom-Lang, K. (1955). Deuterium exchange in proteins and enzymes. *Compt. rend., trav. Lab. Carlsberg Ser. Chim.*, **29,** 385
7. Hellgren, L. and Larsson, K. (1974). On the effect of urea on human epidermis. *Dermatologica*, **149,** 289
8. Montagna, W. (1962). The structure and function of the skin (New York: Academic Press)
9. Allenby, A. C., Creasey, N. H., Edginton, J. A. G., Fletcher, J. A. and Schock, C. (1969). Mechanism of action of accelerants on skin penetration. *Br. J. Dermatol.*, **81,** Suppl. 4, 47

20
Efficacy of a Skin Cream Containing Pyrrolidone Carboxylic Acid in Reducing the Incidence of Subclinical Dry Skin

J. D. MIDDLETON and M. E. ROBERTS

INTRODUCTION

In this paper, the term sub-clinical dry skin is used to describe the very common condition of dry, flaky or chapped skin that occurs particularly in winter. The condition is rarely of sufficient severity to warrant a visit to the doctor or dermatologist, but is sufficiently aggravating for most women to seek a skin cream which will reduce the incidence of dryness, particularly on the hands or face.

There are many products frequently sold under the name of skin moisturizers, that make claims to reduce the incidence of dry skin. The objective of the work reported in this paper was to investigate the efficacy of a formulation containing the sodium salt of pyrrolidone carboxylic acid (PCA). PCA is a normal constituent of stratum corneum and is one of the hygroscopic components of the water-soluble fraction that helps to maintain the moisture content of the corneum[1].

In the study reported here, the efficacy of the PCA cream has been compared with that of a control cream with the same basic formulation, but containing no PCA. For comparative purposes, a third cream, which is widely advertised as being effective in reducing dry skin, was also investigated. The efficacy of the 3 creams was compared in a consumer trial in which 150 women each used the 3 creams consecutively for periods of 2 weeks. The degree of dry skin on their hands was evaluated by trained assessors.

METHODOLOGY

Skin assessment procedure

The degree of skin dryness, flaking or cracking was assessed by trained technicians using a visual numerical scoring technique[2,3].

For assessment, each hand was divided into the following 6 areas: back of hand, thumb web, finger webs, back of fingers, palm and front of fingers. At each assessment, an assessor scored each of the above areas according to the following scheme:

0 = No relevant visible damage
1 = Slight dryness
2 = Marked dryness and/or slight flaking
3 = Severe dryness and/or marked flaking
4 = Severe flaking/slight cracking
6 = Severe cracking

The scores for the 12 areas on each panellist were summed to give a total hand score. The panel of volunteers was divided into 2 halves. Each half saw a different assessor and remained with that assessor throughout the trial. At the end of the trial, the results of the 2 assessors were combined for statistical analysis.

Hand creams

The 3 hand creams were coded as follows:
T = test cream with PCA*
C = control cream, as T but with no PCA
X = cream claiming to be effective

Experimental protocol

One hundred and fifty women, with existing dry or flaky skin on their hands were recruited and the degree of dryness and flakiness assessed by the numerical scoring system. They were divided into six groups in such a way that the mean and range of hand scores in each group were approximately the same. This process was carried out separately for the panellists seeing each of the 2 assessors. Each of the 6 groups was given the hand creams to use at home in one of the possible sequences. Each cream was used for a period of 2 weeks and the degree of hand skin dryness was assessed after using each cream.

* ACO Fukträm, ACO Läkemedel AB, Solna, Sweden.

The creams were referred to by code numbers and letters throughout the trial. Panellists were unaware of the nature of the creams they were using and assessors did not know which creams the panellists had been using.

RESULTS

Table 20.1 shows the mean total hand scores for the six groups using the creams in the six possible sequences. There is a considerable variation in the changes that occurred during the trial and it is difficult to see the effects of the hand creams.

Table 20.1   Mean total hand scores

Cream sequence	No. of panellists	1	2	3	4
			Visit No.		
TCX	24	11.4	11.1	11.8	11.5
TXC	24	12.7	14.1	10.6	15.3
CTX	24	11.5	12.8	11.7	13.8
CXT	23	11.2	13.4	12.2	13.5
XTC	27	12.3	13.2	11.9	16.7
XCT	26	12.5	13.8	14.9	15.6

Table 20.2   Mean changes in total hand score

Cream	1	2	3	Cream mean
		Period No.		
T	0.5	−1.2	1.0	0.11
C	1.7	0.9	4.8	2.47
X	1.1	−2.3	0.9	−0.07
Period Mean	1.1	−0.9	2.3	

Difference between creams required for statistical significance ($p = 0.05$) = 1.56.

Table 20.2 shows the mean changes in total hand score for each cream after each period of use. Because the trial was balanced in terms of initial hand scores and because all possible sequences of cream usage were involved, it is reasonable to calculate mean changes for each period and each cream during the trial. Statistical evaluation of differences between the means for each cream can then determine whether there is any statistically significant difference between the creams.

The difference between creams required for statistical significance between creams as determined by analysis of variance is also shown in Table 20.2.

The statistical calculations show that the cream containing PCA (coded T) resulted in a lower degree of skin dryness and flaking than the control cream without PCA (coded C). There was no significant difference between the PCA

179

cream and the cream which is advertised as being effective (coded X). Cream X was also more effective than the control cream.

The results show that creams containing hygroscopic ingredients such as PCA can reduce the incidence of dry and flaky skin under normal use conditions.

References

1. Laden, K. and Spitzer, R. J. (1967). Identification of a natural moisturising agent in skin. *J. Soc. Cosmet. Chem.*, **18,** 351
2. Gibsòn, I. M. (1973). The evaluation of hand care preparations. *J. Soc. Cosmet. Chem.*, **24,** 31
3. Middleton, J. D. (1974). Development of a skin cream designed to reduce dry and flaky skin. *J. Soc. Cosmet. Chem.*, **25,** 519

21
Ichthyosiform Erythroderma. 10 Years Treatment with Retinoic Acid

J. A. MILNE

PATIENT AND METHODS

Following the publications of Stüttgen[1] and Beer[2] on the use of vitamin A acid in the treatment of ichthyosiform erythroderma, Thomson and Milne[3] reported the treatment of a seven-year-old girl with ichthyosiform erythroderma (epidermolytic hyperkeratosis) (Figure 21.1) by topical and systemic retinoic acid.

Retinoic acid 0.1% in yellow soft paraffin was used topically or alternatively systemically, administered as 16 mg capsules to a calculated equivalent dose of 50 000 I.U. of retinol/daily. When 0.1% retinoic acid in yellow soft paraffin was applied topically there was marked clinical improvment in the area treated. When administered systemically (1 × 16 mg t.i.d.) there was dramatic clinical improvement of all lesions with virtual complete control of the excessive keratinization although some underlying erythema remained (Figure 21.2). No significant improvement was seen with topically applied soft yellow paraffin, or equivalent doses of retinol or retinal.

The patient was maintained on systemic therapy for 3 years during which time her skin remained well. Regular monitoring of liver function and ophthalmic examinations failed to reveal any evidence of hypervitaminosis A or visual defect. The menarche occurred at age 12 with a regular cycle and normal flow. At the age of 14 the patient developed personality changes, becoming aggressive and refusing to treat her skin either topically or systemically. These symptoms have persisted and therapy is now intermittent. When retinoic acid is applied topically or taken systemically the skin still

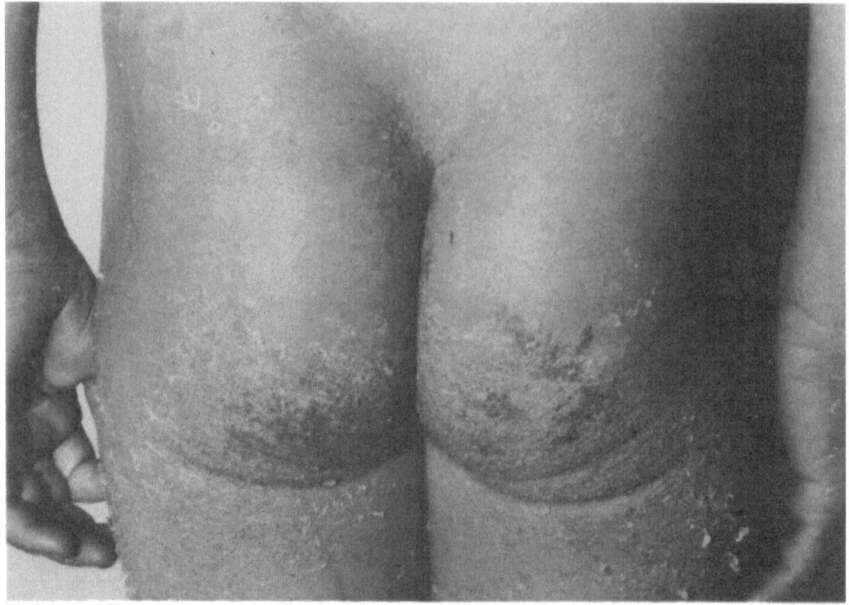

Figure 21.1   Lesions of buttock before therapy

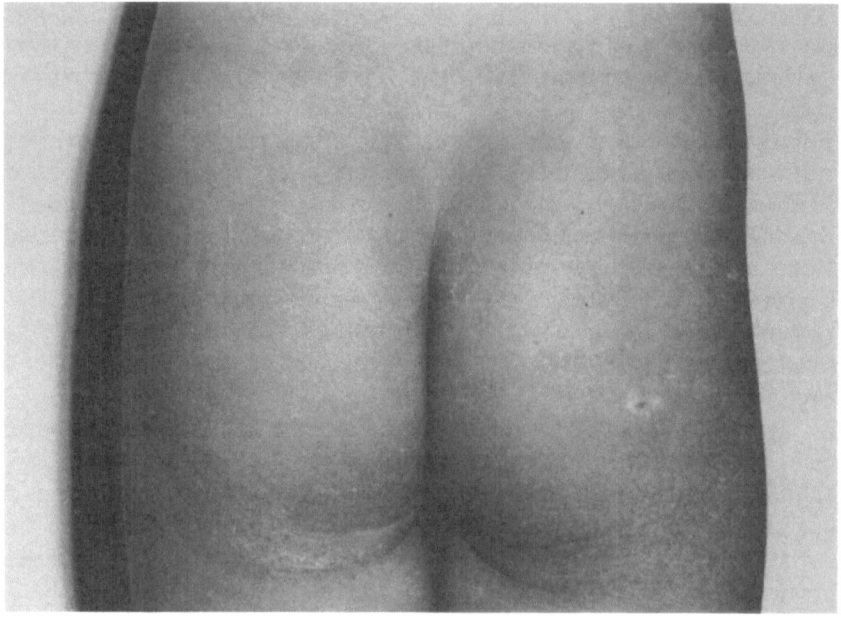

Figure 21.2   Lesions of buttock 2 months after commencement of systemic therapy

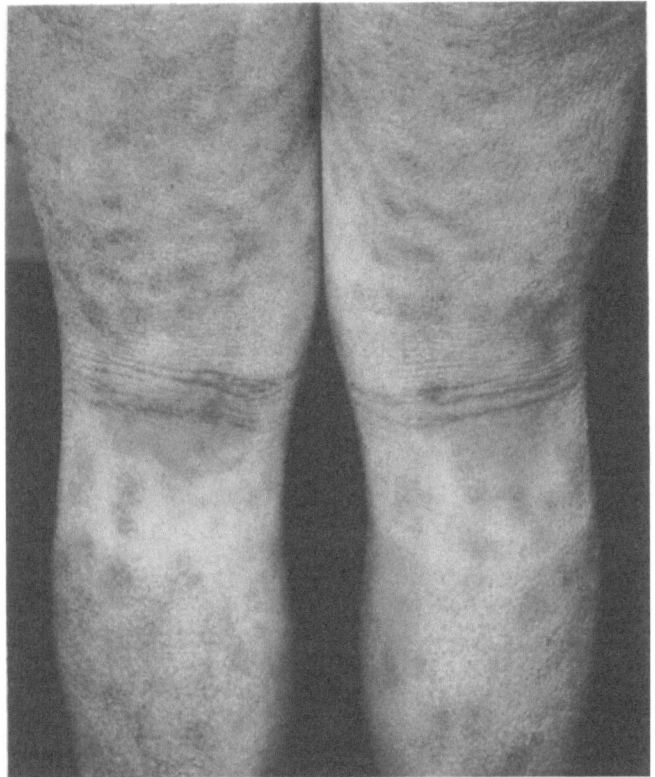

Figure 21.3   Present condition of skin, age 17. No therapy for 6 months

rapidly clears. At present she has had no therapy for 6 months and her skin lesions have relapsed (Figure 21.3).

One problem throughout this patient's treatment has been the fall in potency of the retinoic acid, within about 4–8 weeks of obtaining it from the manufacturer. While there is no doubt that retinoic acid, either topically or systemically, controls the excessive keratinization of this disorder, relapse is rapid on withdrawal of treatment.

References

1. Stüttgen, V. G. (1962). Zur Lokalbehandlung Von Keratosen Mit Vitamin-A-Säure. *Dermatologica*, **124**, 65
2. Beer, P. (1962). Untersuchungen über die Wirkung der Vitamin-A-Säure. *Dermatologica*, **124**, 192
3. Thomson, J. and Milne, J. A. (1969). The use of retinoic acid in congenital ichthyosiform erythroderma. *Br. J. Dermatol.*, **81**, 452

22
Aspects of Long-Term Treatment of Ichthyotic Dermatoses with Vitamin A Acid

G. STÜTTGEN and W. SCHALLA

INTRODUCTION

Oral or topical vitamin A acid has therapeutic value in the treatment of pathological keratinization expressed as scaling and follicular keratoses as occurring in ichthyosiform dermatoses (Stüttgen[1,2]).

Pharmacokinetic investigations of vitamin A acid have demonstrated that both oral and local therapy can be used. Schaefer and Zesch[3] have shown that the concentration of vitamin A acid in the transition area from epidermis to corium, after local application of a 0.1% preparation, is 10 μM or 3 μg/g tissue. The clinical effect resulting from such an application corresponds to that achieved by oral administration of 100 mg vitamin A acid.

PATIENTS AND METHODS

The toxic dosage determined by Kretzschmar and Leuschner[4] in animal experiments was confirmed in our clinical investigations with patients. Oral doses of 50 to 120 mg vitamin A acid daily cause side-effects, such as severe headaches, dryness of the lips, etc. (Table 22.1). However, a dose of 10 to 20 mg is well tolerated by most patients. The clinically visible side-effects encountered with oral vitamin A acid at doses of 100 mg correspond to those observed with high doses of vitamin A palmitate.

Table 22.1   Side effects after oral vitamin A acid (50–200 mg daily/4 weeks) in 30 patients

Side effect	Frequency
Dryness of lips	24
Headache	23
Flushing	22
Dryness of skin	15
Tiredness	13
Bulb-pressure sensitivity	11
Loss of appetite	11
Increased thirst	9
Nausea	8
Pruritus increased	7
Pruritus diminished	4
Dizziness	6
Increased sweating	6
Petechial eruptions	5
Dandruff	4
Oedema of the face	3 (100–200 mg)
Changes in the psychological state	3 (100–200 mg)
Dryness of the mucous membrane of the nose	3
Alopecia diffusa	2
Unconsciousness with complete reversibility after 4 days 100 mg/daily	2 (200 mg)

The local application of 0.1% ointment frequently causes local skin irritation in the form of reddening, oedema, itching and scaling. On the other hand erythema and oedema very rarely develop after oral vitamin A acid therapy — and then only with high doses above 100 mg. There is no doubt that oral administration of vitamin A acid can replace local therapy. The dosage required for the initial therapy is high in the first few weeks, until first signs of improvement of the ichthyosiform dermatoses are visible. In cases of congenital ichthyosiform erythroderma we were able to achieve a definite improvement with pronounced decrease in scaling by a dosage of 20 to 60 mg daily. After improvement and loosening of horny patches it was possible to maintain the improved state of the skin with 20 mg twice daily. (It should be noted that the dosage given here refers to adults and is to be proportionally reduced in children.) The treatment of ichthyosis vulgaris requires approximately the same dosage of vitamin A acid as for therapy of ichthyosiform erythroderma. The effect of oral treatment in one patient is shown in Figure 22.1.

In cases of Darier's disease a relatively high initial dose of at least 100 mg vitamin A acid daily is necessary in order to achieve a sufficient therapeutic effect in patients with extensive skin lesions. Side-effects (Table 22.1) were reduced by palliative treatment and by early reduction to maintenance dose levels. The dosage was reduced every 7 to 10 days by 20 mg. The maintenance dose in Darier's disease was 20 mg twice daily. Further lowering of this dosage was followed by a relapse. The management of the skin condition in the

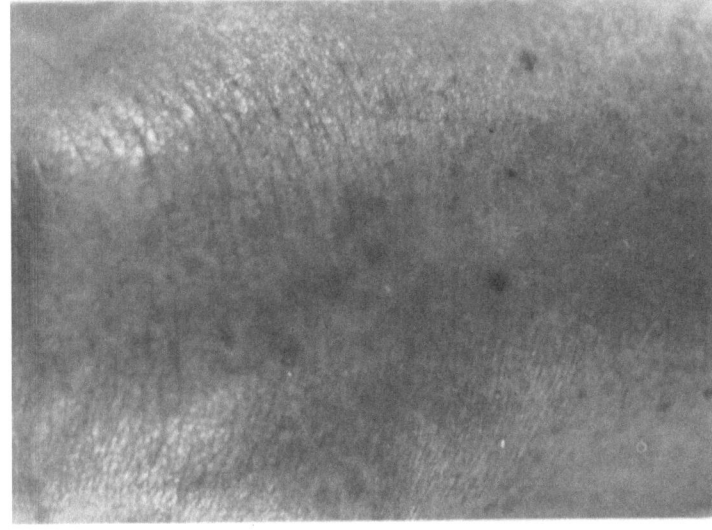

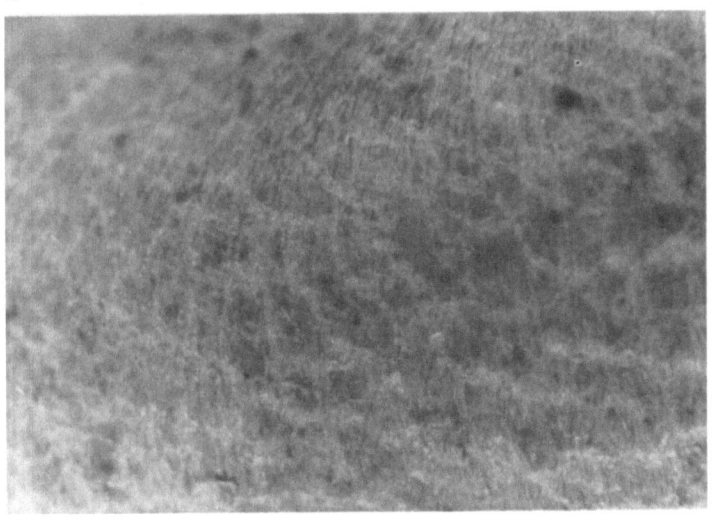

Figure 22.1 Ichthyosis congenita before (a) and after (b) oral treatment with 60 mg vitamin A acid (male, 54 years old, upper arm)

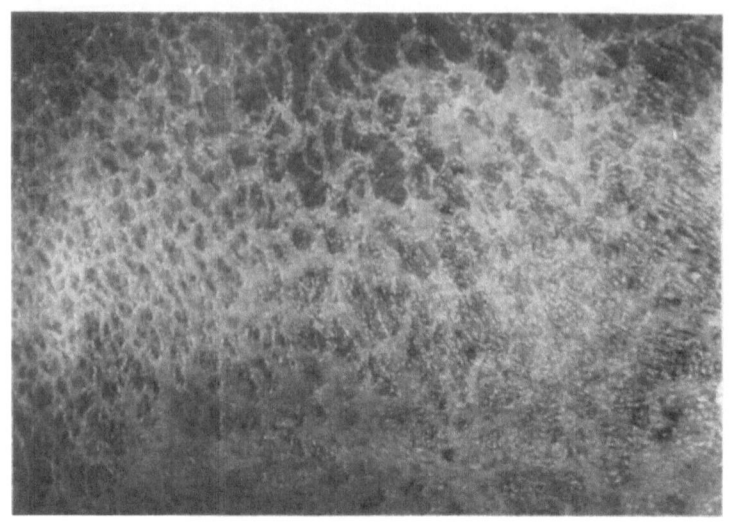

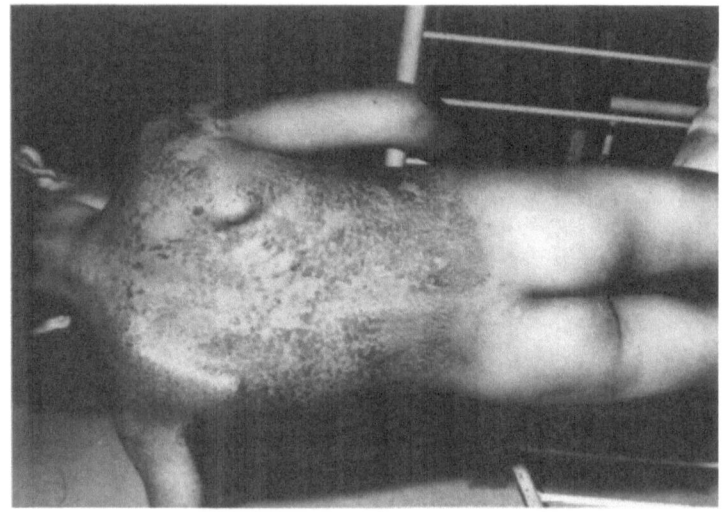

a

188

d

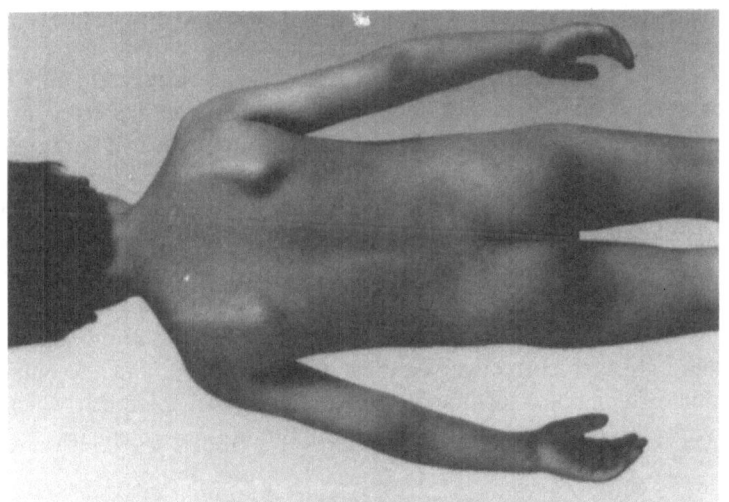

c

Figure 22.2 Ichthyosis vulgaris before (a) (b) and after (c) (d), combined therapy for 6 weeks. Local treatment was with 0.1% vitamin A acid ointment for 2 weeks followed by 0.05% for a further 2 weeks with a subsequent concentration of 0.01%. After 2 weeks topical treatment, oral therapy was started. This consisted of 5 mg, twice daily for 3 weeks followed by 5 mg daily

ichthyoses and in Darier's disease depends to some extent on climate and this has to be taken into account.

We have observed that for the initiation of effective therapy, 50 to 100 mg have to be administered orally which is at the upper limit of toxic effects as mentioned above. In the last 2 years, we have treated patients for 2 weeks with local 0.1% vitamin A acid until this treatment becomes irritant and then we commence oral treatment. The oral dosage can be reduced to about 20 mg twice daily and after 4 weeks to about 10 mg twice daily. Simultaneously, local treatment can be reduced below the development of irritancy by application of 0.05% vitamin A acid ointment and in some cases we can reduce the vitamin A acid concentration in the ointment to 0.01% (Figure 22.2). Thus the side effects of local and oral therapy can be avoided by combination of both types of treatment which suggests that in the future when programming the therapy of ichthyotic patients, the combination of local and oral therapy should be considered. When we have stopped oral therapy and tried to initiate a maintenance treatment with local vitamin A acid at low concentrations, relapses occur within 2 months. After the re-appearance of ichthyotic lesions, oral administration of vitamin A acid at the lower dose was repeated with satisfactory results.

COMMENTS

The therapy of ichthyotic dermatoses has to be lifelong. Our schedule allows for the application of minimal amount of vitamin A acid without any adverse reactions in the skin. In our 5 years experience we have observed in only one case minor toxic reactions with a high dosage which was expressed in an abnormal high serum level of liver enzymes. These values returned to normal 4 weeks after reduction of the dosage. Intermittent oral vitamin A acid given at intervals of about 2 months seems to cause changes in the intercellular matrix and terminal vessels. These effects have been verified by electron microscopy and may be caused by changes in the mesenchymal epidermal interactions which influence the development of ichthyoses[5,6]. However, we need further observations concerning the target site of vitamin A acid before one can evaluate these changes correctly. We think that we have found the optimal dose schedule of combined local and oral vitamin A acid treatment which is effective over years at a low dosage level without prominent side-effects.

References

1. Stüttgen, G. (1962). Zur Lokalbehandlung von Keratosen mit Vitamin-A-Säure. *Dermatologica (Basel)*, **124**, 65
2. Stüttgen, G. (1975). Oral vitamin A acid therapy. *Acta Dermato-Venereol. (Stockh.)*, *Suppl.*, **74**, 174

3. Schaefer, H. and Zesch, A. (1975). Penetration of vitamin A acid into human skin. *Acta Dermato-Venereol. (Stockh), Suppl.*, **74,** 50

4. Kretzschmar, R. and Leuschner, F. (1975). Biosynthesis and metabolism of retinoic acid. *Acta Dermato-Venereol. (Stockh.) Suppl.*, **74,** 25

5. Wolff, H. H., Christophers, E. and Braun-Falco, O. (1970). Changes in epidermal differentiation after vitamin A acid. An electron microscopic study. *Arch. Klin. Exp. Dermatol.*, **237,** 774

6. Merker, M. and Stüttgen, G. (1975). Electron microscope findings after toxic doses of vitamin A acid in man. *Acta Dermato-Venereol. (Stockh.) Suppl.*, **74,** 64

23
Treatment of Disorders of Keratinization with an Oral Stereoisomer of Retinoic Acid

G. L. PECK and F. W. YODER

ABSTRACT

Fifty-four patients with treatment-resistant disorders of keratinization were treated with oral 13-cis retinoic acid, a synthetic stereoisomer of retinoic acid, for one to 29 weeks. The dosage varied from 0.5 to 6.0 mg/kg/day. The median patient dosage was 2 mg/kg daily for 8 weeks. Excellent responses have been observed in patients with congenital ichthyosiform erythroderma, lamellar ichthyosis, Darier's disease, and pityriasis rubra pilaris. However, patients with epidermolytic hyperkeratosis have responded only partially, and patients with psoriasis, nevus comedonicus, X-linked ichthyosis, and Netherton's syndrome have either not responded or have worsened. Commonly observed side effects included cheilitis, facial dermatitis, xerosis, skin fragility, and conjunctivitis. The erythrocyte sedimentation rate was elevated in 7 patients; no other abnormal laboratory tests, including liver function tests, were noted in this group of patients. The mechanism by which this synthetic retinoid alters these disease states is not clear but may be related to the observed ability of vitamin A to affect glycoprotein synthesis and epithelial differentiation. Our results indicate that synthetic retinoids, such as 13-cis retinoic acid, may represent a potent new class of drugs in the treatment of cutaneous disease.

INTRODUCTION

Vitamin A, and more recently retinoic acid (all-trans vitamin A acid) has long been used either systemically or topically in the treatment of keratinizing disorders of the skin[1]. The therapeutic responses have been inconsistent and limited by either systemic toxicity, or local irritation when applied topically. Retinoic acid has proven to be more potent than vitamin A in the treatment of these conditions. However, the hypervitaminosis A syndrome induced by systemic retinoic acid has prompted the search for synthetic derivatives with similar or greater therapeutic activity but lower toxicity. Preliminary data in animals and man have indicated that 13-cis retinoic acid[2,3] may be less toxic than the naturally occurring all-trans retinoic acid[4], and was therefore selected for testing in this study.

MATERIALS AND METHODS

Drugs

13-cis retinoic acid (RO-43780, Hoffman–La Roche, Nutley, New Jersey) was administered in 10 mg and 20 mg capsules.

Patients

Fifty-four patients with chronic, treatment-resistant, keratinizing dermatoses were included in this study. The diagnoses were based on typical clinical histories, physical examinations, and biopsies of diseased skin. The 7 patients with congenital lamellar ichthyosis had the characteristic large brown centrally adherent scale with minimal underlying erythema. The 2 patients, a brother and sister who we prefer to designate non-bullous congenital ichthyosiform erythroderma, were distinguished from lamellar ichthyosis by the presence of erythroderma, fine white loosely adherent scale, and marked parakeratosis histologically. All had responded poorly to standard topical keratolytics and emollients. Several of these patients had received topical α-hydroxy acids and topical retinoic acid with partial improvement.

Patients with recalcitrant Darier's disease were often complicated by bacterial infection. Therapy with methotrexate, topical retinoic acid, or oral vitamin A (up to 500 000 I.U. per day for 2 years) were ineffective. Four patients had responded to deep split thickness excision of diseased skin in localized areas[5,6].

The patients with pityriasis rubra pilaris had not responded to topical retinoic acid, oral vitamin A (750 000 I.U. for 6 weeks), topical keratolytics, topical α-hydroxy acids, or systemic methotrexate.

Treatment with 13-cis retinoic acid was usually begun at a minimum dosage of 1 mg/kg/day given in divided daily doses. Dosage was increased at 2- to 3-week intervals until significant therapeutic benefit or toxicity was noted. Treatment was stopped after 4 months and was resumed in responsive patients after a 2-month interval.

Application of hydrophilic ointment was permitted in those patients who required a topical lubricant. Hydroxyzine hydrochloride was given to a few patients for control of pruritus. White petrolatum was used for the cheilitis resulting from treatment with 13-cis retinoic acid. Oral erythromycin or cloxacillin was necessary to control the recurrent cutaneous infections of 2 patients with Darier's disease and the one with nevus comedonicus.

Laboratory examinations taken at 2-week intervals included a urinalysis and blood studies for uric acid, calcium, phosphorus, SGOT, SGPT, alkaline phosphatase, lactic dehydrogenase, total bilirubin, total protein, albumin, creatinine, blood urea nitrogen, glucose, electrolytes, carotene, vitamin A, haemoglobin, haematocrit, white blood count, platelet count, prothrombin time, partial thromboplastin time, and erythrocyte sedimentation rate.

RESULTS

Clinical results

Excellent improvement was seen in congenital ichthyosiform erythroderma, lamellar ichthyosis (Figures 23.1–2), Darier's disease, and in pityriasis rubra pilaris (Figures 23.3–4). Improvement in some of these patients was seen within 2 weeks, usually beginning after 2 to 4 days of treatment. Others required higher doses for extended periods (10–12 weeks) before improving. Improvement was characterized by decreased scaling, a decrease in underlying erythema, and a decrease in induration, ultimately giving a normal or near normal appearance on close inspection. In the above diseases the scalp, palms, and soles were less responsive than the other involved areas. Seasonal variation of therapeutic response was noted in the patients with lamellar ichthyosis, who had responded to 13-cis retinoic acid at a dosage of 1 mg/kg/day in the summer but required 2–3 mg/kg/day in the winter. Those patients begun on therapy in the late fall responded only partially. Similarly, patients with pityriasis rubra pilaris responded less well in the winter. However, no seasonal variation was seen in congenital ichthyosiform erythroderma or in Darier's disease. In fact, the 2

Table 23.1 Clinical results

Diagnosis	Response* (number of patients)			
	1+	2+	3+	4+
Lamellar ichthyosis	1	2	1	3
Congenital ichthyosiform erythroderma	–	–	–	2
Darier's disease	1	1	3	3
Pityriasis rubra pilaris	2	1	–	2
Epidermolytic hyperkeratosis	4	–	–	–

* 4+ = >90%, 3+ = >75%, 2+ = >50%, and 1+ = >25% clearing

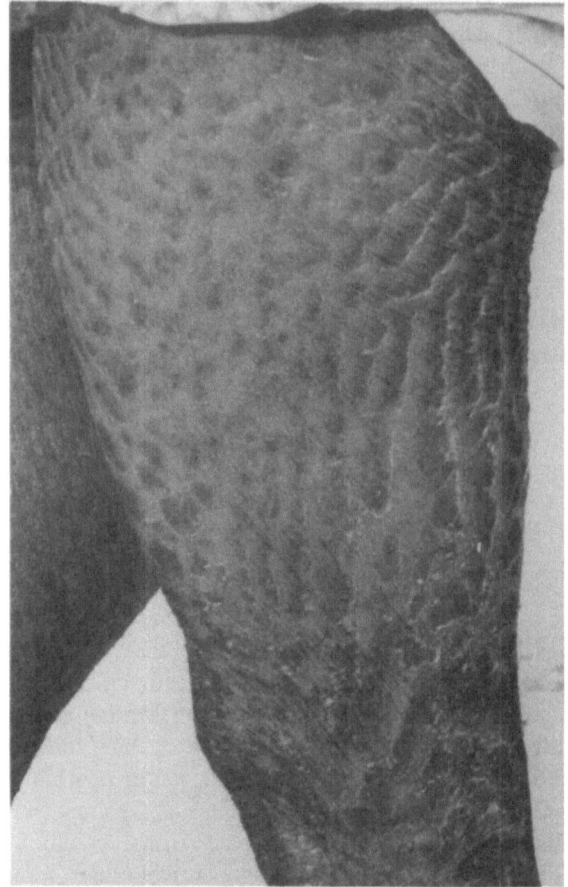

Figure 23.1   Lamellar ichthyosis, lateral thigh, prior to treatment

patients with congenital ichthyosiform erythroderma were well maintained in the winter at a dosage of 1 mg/kg given on alternate days.

All responsive patients relapsed within 2 weeks after discontinuation of therapy at the end of the initial 4-month treatment period, and then responded to readministration of the drug after the 2-month rest period.

The patients with X-linked ichthyosis, Netherton's syndrome, nevus comedonicus, or psoriasis either worsened or failed to improve.

Side effects

Clinical

Cheilitis was noted in 52 of the 54 patients. It was usually mild, appearing early

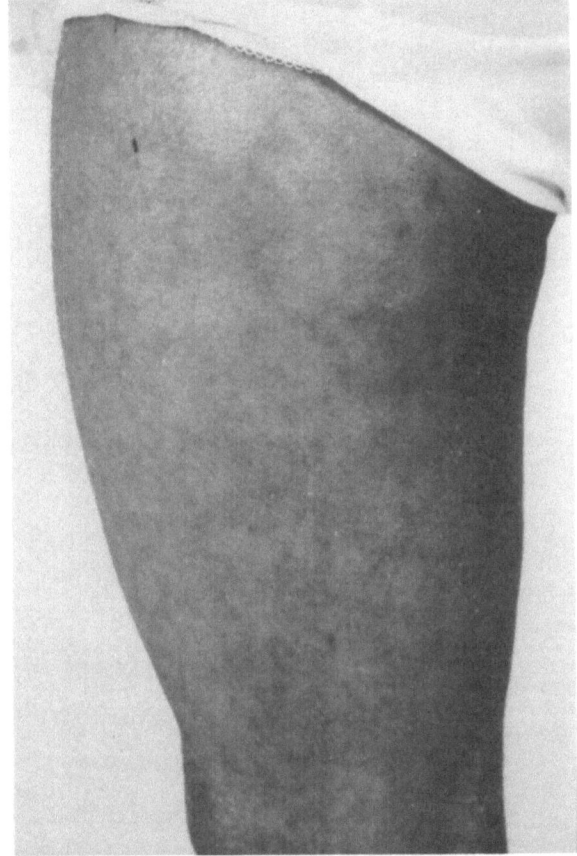

Figure 23.2   After 4 weeks treatment with 120 mg/day 13-cis retinoic acid

in the course of therapy, and was controllable with frequent applications of petrolatum. Facial dermatitis, xerosis, conjunctivitis, and dryness of the nasal mucosa with nosebleed were seen more frequently in the winter (Table 23.2).

Laboratory

The erythrocyte sedimentation rate was elevated in 7 patients. No other abnormal laboratory test, including liver function tests, were observed in this group of patients.

DISCUSSION

The results from this and our previous studies[7-9] indicate that short-term treatment with 13-cis retinoic acid is a safe and effective treatment for several

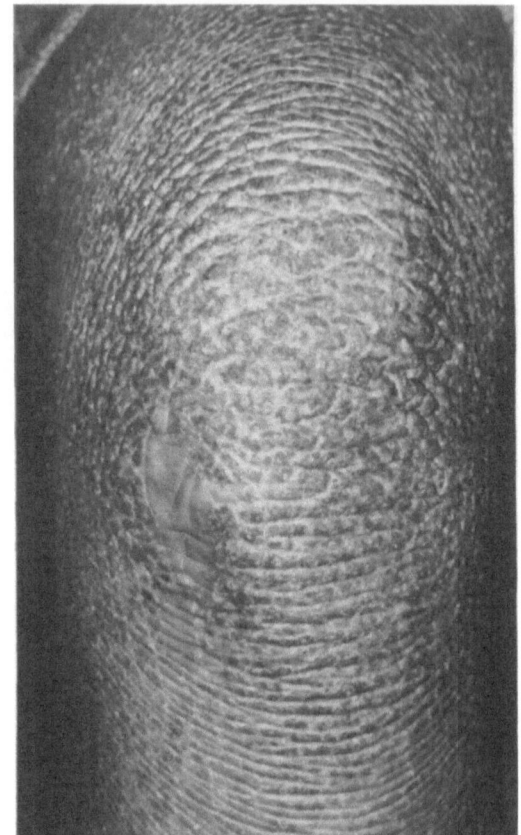

Figure 23.3   Pityriasis rubra pilaris, knee, prior to treatment

Table 23.2   Side effects in 54 patients

Cheilitis	52
Facial dermatitis	15
Conjunctivitis	11
Skin fragility	9
Dry skin	12
Increased pruritus	3
Dryness of nasal mucosa	6
Nosebleed	4
Headache	5
Increased appetite	4
Decreased appetite	2
Arthralgia	2
Fatigue	2
Finger tip peeling	1
Allergic skin reaction (paraben sensitivity?)	1
Elevation of erythrocyte sedimentation rate	7

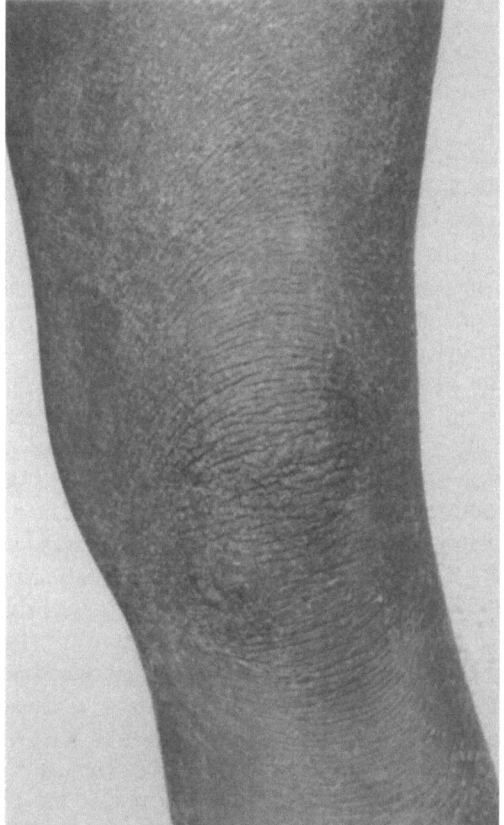

Figure 23.4   After 11 weeks treatment with 160 mg/day 13-cis retinoic acid

dermatologic disorders of keratinization. The lack of a therapeutic response in psoriasis, X-linked ichthyosis, Netherton's syndrome, and nevus comedonicus in this report suggests that the mode of action of this agent may be highly specific.

Successful treatment of congenital ichthyosiform erythroderma, pityriasis rubra pilaris, and Darier's disease have been documented with oral all-trans retinoic acid in daily doses varying from 10 to 60 mg for several weeks to months[10-12]. Orfanos et al. used oral 13-cis retinoic acid in the treatment of psoriasis with equivocal results[3]. More recently, better results were obtained in psoriasis using a trimethylphenyl derivative of retinoic acid (RO-10/9359, Hoffman–La Roche, Basle), up to 100 mg/day, either alone[13] or in combination with topical dithranol[14]. Since this derivative appears to be more effective than 13-cis retinoic acid in the treatment of psoriasis, a study comparing these two synthetic retinoids in the treatment of other disorders of keratinization should be of value.

The value of using the synthetic retinoids in the treatment of these dermatoses lies not only in the excellent therapeutic response but also in the comparative lack of toxicity. The synthetic analogues, including 13-cis retinoic acid, were developed in an effort to counter the toxicity problems of vitamin A and its naturally occurring derivatives. For example, one advantage of the synthetic retinoids is that, unlike vitamin A, they are not stored in the liver. thus far, liver toxicity has not been observed with the use of these synthetic agents[15]. In contrast to the documented toxicity of oral all-trans retinoic acid, we have failed to observe in our series of patients bulb pressure sensitivity, enhanced thirst, nausea, dizziness, petechiae, dandruff, psychological changes, diffuse alopecia, or unconsciousness[4]. The chronic toxicity of 13-cis retinoic acid remains to be determined.

The mechanism of action of 13-cis retinoic acid in normal and diseased human skin has not been studied. Many biological effects of vitamin A, especially its ability to labilize biological membranes and release lysosomal enzymes, have been described in detail[16]. Vitamin A and its derivatives control cell growth and differentiation in epithelial tissues. Retinoic acid, in particular, is a potent stimulator of mitosis in the epidermis[17]. Excess vitamin A and its derivatives also have been demonstrated to inhibit keratinization and induce a mucous metaplasia with enhanced glycoprotein synthesis in several laboratory models, such as embryonic chick skin in organ culture[18,19]. The mode of action of topical retinoic acid in acne is thought to be the increased production of non-adherent surface scales, which prevents follicular occlusion and comedo formation[20]. None of the known effects, however, can fully explain the apparent disease and individual specificity of the clinical response to 13-cis retinoic acid nor do they explain its ability to reduce the erythema in these diseases.

The results of this study, in which a synthetic retinoid was found to have a profound beneficial effect in the treatment of disorders of keratinization, should be of importance to areas other than dermatology. For instance, preneoplastic squamous metaplasia of tracheo-bronchial and urinary bladder epithelia may be other keratinizing disorders of man that could be successfully treated with the synthetic retinoids, as suggested by Sporn[15,21]. Finally, patients with these cutaneous diseases, which have responded to 13-cis retinoic acid, may provide useful information in the evaluation of newer and potentially more potent and less toxic synthetic retinoids.

References

1. De Bersaques, J. (1972). Topical vitamin A acid. *Arch. Belg. Dermatol. Syph.*, **28**, 315
2. Hoffman–La Roche Investigational Drug Brochure RO-43780, 13-cis Retinoic Acid, August 28, 1972
3. Orfanos, C. E., Schmidt, H, W., Mahrle, G. and Runne, U., Koln: Die Wirksamkeit von Vitamin A-Saure (VAS) bei Psoriasis. Ortliche Kombinationsbehandlung mit Corticoiden.

Zwei neue VAS-Praparate zur peroralen Therapie. (1972). *Arch. Dermatol. Forsch.*, **244,** 424

4. Stuttgen, G. (1975). Oral vitamin A acid therapy. *Acta Derm. Venereol. (Stockh.)*, **55,** (*Suppl.* 74), 174
5. Cohen, I. K., Kraemer, K. H. and Peck, G. L. (1976). Cornifying Darier disease — a unique variant. *Arch. Dermatol.*, **112,** 504
6. Dellon, A. L., Chretien, P. B. and Peck, G. L. (1977). Successful treatment of Darier's disease by partial-thickness removal of skin. *Plastic and Reconstructive Surgery.* **59,** 823
7. Peck, G. L. and Yoder, F. W. (1976). Treatment of lamellar ichthyosis and other keratinising dermatoses with an oral synthetic retinoid. *Lancet*, **ii,** 1172
8. Yoder, F. W. and Peck, G. L. (1976). Treatment of keratinizing dermatoses with oral 13-cis retinoic acid. *Clin. Res.*, **24,** 624A
9. Yoder, F. W. and Peck, G. L. (1977). Treatment of lamellar ichthyosis, Darier's disease, and pityriasis rubra pilaris with oral 13-cis retinoic acid. *Clin. Res.* **25,** 288A
10. Thomson, J. and Milne, J. A. (1969). The use of retinoic acid in congenital ichthyosiform erythroderma. *Br. J. Dermatol.*, **81,** 452
11. Eriksen, L. and Cormane, R. H. (1975). Oral retinoic acid as therapy for congenital ichthyosiform erythroderma. *Br. J. Dermatol.*, **92,** 343
12. Gunther, S. (1976). Vitamin A acid: Clinical investigations with 405 patients. *Cutis*, **17,** 287
13. Ott, F. and Bollag, W. (1975). Therapie der psoriasis mit einem oral Wirksamen Neuen Vitamin-A-Saure Derivat. *Schweiz. med. Wschr.*, **105,** 439
14. Orfanos, C. E., and Runne, U. (1976). Systemic use of a new retinoid with and without local dithranol treatment in generalized psoriasis. *Br. J. Dermatol.*, **95,** 101
15. Sporn, M. B., Dunlop, N. M., Newton, D. L. and Smith, J. M. (1976). Prevention of chemical carcinogenesis by vitamin A and its synthetic analogs (retinoids). *Fed. Proc.*, **35,** 1332
16. Zbinden, G. (1975). Pharmacology of vitamin A acid (β-all-trans retinoic acid). *Acta Derm. Venereol.*, *(Stockh.)*, **55,** (Suppl. 74), 21
17. Christophers, E. and Wolff, H. H. (1975). Effects of vitamin A acid in skin: In vivo and in vitro studies. Ibid. **55,** (Suppl. 74), 42
18. Peck, G. L., Elias, P. M. and Wetzel, B. (1977). Influence of vitamin A on differentiating epithelia. In M. Seiji and I. A. Bernstein (eds.) *Biochemistry of Cutaneous Epidermal Differentiation* (Tokyo: University of Tokyo Press) pp 110–126
19. Wilkoff, L. J., Peckham, J. C., Dulmadge, E. A. and Mowry, R. W. (1976). Evaluation of vitamin A analogs in modulating epithelial differentiation of 13-day chick embryo metatarsal skin explants. *Cancer Research* **36,** 964
20. Fulton, J. E. (1975). Vitamin A acid   The last five years. *J. Cut. Path.*, **2,** 155
21. Sporn, M. B., Squire, R. A., Brown, C. C., Smith, J. M., Wenk, M. L. and Springer, S. (1977). 13-cis-retinoic acid: inhibition of bladder carcinogenesis in the rat. *Science*, **195,** 487

Index